Making Sense of Spirituality in

DATE DUE

For my wife Mandy and children Stacey and Matthew, in recognition of all their love and support

For Churchill Livingstone:

Senior Commissioning Editor: Jacqueline Curthoys
Project Manager: Gail Murray
Project Development Manager: Katrina Mather
Designer: George Ajayi

Making Sense of Spirituality in Nursing Practice
An Interactive Approach

Wilfred McSherry BSc(Hons) MPhil PCGE(FE) RGN NT
Lecturer in Adult Nursing, Department of Health Studies,
University of York, York, UK

Foreword by

Keith Cash BA(Hons) MSc PhD RGN RMN
Professor of Nursing, Leeds Metropolitan University, Leeds, UK

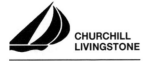
CHURCHILL
LIVINGSTONE

EDINBURGH LONDON NEW YORK PHILADELPHIA ST LOUIS SYDNEY TORONTO 2000

CHURCHILL LIVINGSTONE
An imprint of Harcourt Publishers Limited

© Harcourt Publishers Limited 2000

 is a registered trademark of Harcourt Publishers Limited

The right of Wilfred McSherry to be identified as author of this work
has been asserted by him in accordance with the Copyright, Designs
and Patents Act 1988

First published 2000

ISBN 0 443 06356 7

British Library Cataloguing in Publication Data
A catalogue record for this book is available from the British Library

Library of Congress Cataloging in Publication Data
A catalog record for this book is available from the Library of
Congress

Note
Medical knowledge is constantly changing. As new information
becomes available, changes in treatment, procedures, equipment and
the use of drugs become necessary. The author and the publishers
have, as far as it is possible, taken care to ensure that the information
given in this text is accurate and up to date. However, readers are
strongly advised to confirm that the information, especially with
regard to drug usage, complies with the latest legislation and
standards of practice.

The
publisher's
policy is to use
**paper manufactured
from sustainable forests**

Printed in China

Contents

Foreword

Spirituality is a notoriously difficult concept to teach and to learn about. It is especially difficult for someone like me who is agnostic. This is because some of the spiritual experiences that people report are foreign to me, although some are familiar. I think that it is also difficult nowadays for those people who do have some sense of a spiritual life. Nurses face very strong pressures today to work in certain ways. There are contradictory messages that they have to listen to and to answer. The first message is that they should base everything that they do on evidence, on research and therefore on a scientific view of the world. The second is that they should see the patient as a consumer of their services. The third is the message from patients that they wish to be seen as individuals, with the deep respect for their beliefs that this entails.

It is not clear that these positions are compatible. Treating patients as consumers means that they are such, as recipients of services that have been paid for, but this does not mean that the person providing the service has to respect them. It is possible to be a manager without having any understanding of, for example, the spiritual needs of one's customers.

Nurses, however, have to deal with the most personal and intimate details of a person's life. They are able to do things to a person's body that lay people regard as shocking or bizarre. They have to deal with people who are having the most profound personal experiences – confronting (or not) their own mortality, the end of those to whom they are closest, the birth of a person, and pain and distress, physical and mental. How they do this and how well they do it depends on certain factors.

The first is the amount of care and compassion that they can offer. While it is necessary to be technically proficient and efficient, this is not sufficient for good nursing. There are skills that are not just technical but are to do with the sensitivity and human qualities that nurses bring to their work. This becomes even more the case as we move towards an increasingly secular, multicultural country. There are now many belief systems that nurses have to deal with. The decline of organized Christianity means that the assumption that the majority of patients will have a systematic view of Christianity is no longer reasonable. There is an increasing number of patients with Muslim, Hindu, Buddhist and other beliefs, where the religion is not just a creed but strongly associated with the person's daily life. The complexity of beliefs that now face the nurse is pronounced. To meet the needs of patients, therefore, it is necessary not just to have knowledge of, for example, the dietary codes of certain religions, important though these are, but also the willingness, openness and the skills to be able to address new beliefs and customs.

An example from my own experience illustrates the point. Many years ago I worked with a charge nurse who believed that all Muslims were vegetarian. Because of this belief, a patient who was bed-bound lived on an unremitting diet of pizza because the hospital kitchen thought that all vegetarians ate pizza. Elementary errors were made about the dietary customs of a particular religious group, and also incorrect assumptions were made about a (possibly) non-religious belief system, vegetarianism. The patient concerned had a miserable and confusing experience. There was a lack of knowledge and there was a lack of care because there was no attempt to find out what the patient really wanted. The moral stance that sees it as important to examine a patient's beliefs in order to deliver culturally sensitive care was missing.

Today, this would be regarded as unacceptable because there is a rhetoric of holism. Every nurse is now taught that a holistic view of the patient is required; however, to develop the emotional and theoretical sensitivity and practical skills necessary to work in a holistic way is difficult. This is why I welcome this book by Wilf McSherry. It provides a clear direction through the theoretical muddle that exists around the use of the term 'spirituality' in nursing. Importantly, it shows how the term can be incorporated into nursing practice, both theoretically and practically. But of prime importance is that it provides the exercises that will enable the student reader to develop the ability to meet these beliefs with sensitivity, and deliver the nursing care that is required.

Keith Cash

Preface

The aim of this book is to provide a practical interactive resource for students and qualified nurses who seek an introduction into the spiritual dimension of nursing. Therefore I have written in a style and language that facilitate reflection and learning, drawing on relevant literature, which is referenced within the text.

This book reflects my experiences as a practitioner, researcher and educationalist. As a practitioner, I offer case studies, some of which I personally encountered while in practice. (To protect patient anonymity, names and some particulars have been changed.) These case studies are used to relate some of the abstract theory to practice and vice versa. By drawing upon my knowledge as a researcher who has investigated and is still investigating this aspect of nursing, I offer an insight that is balanced, relevant and accurate in that it reflects contemporary thought, issues and developments. As an educationalist, I draw upon my classroom experience in making the text interesting, stimulating and challenging. I hope that by combining these three perspectives I have developed a text that will generate a deeper understanding of some important issues surrounding the spiritual dimension of care.

The design of this book is intended to encourage interaction with the material presented. Each chapter contains several activities that require thought and reflection. Combined with the case study material, these activities reinforce the points made and show how theory can be applied to practice. The chapters have been presented in a logical order, progressing from an examination of the spiritual heritage of nursing to an exploration of contemporary research and educational issues.

You may well ask yourself why a nurse lecturer should be interested in this aspect of care. It is my firm belief that nurses receive little or no instruction in this very sensitive and personal aspect of our lives. It was with this belief in mind that I decided to investigate spirituality and spiritual care, not only conceptually and theoretically but also clinically and educationally. I am conscious that some of the material presented reflects a Judeo–Christian approach to spirituality. However, this is not a deliberate attempt to exclude other world faiths but is a reflection of my personal experiences. I hope that readers from other world faiths will still find the material relevant, stimulating and challenging. With reference to the concepts of spirituality and spiritual need, these terms may not be universally understood or relevant to all individuals. It would be a grave mistake to assume that everyone who requires nursing care will present with spiritual needs or identify with the concepts discussed.

Ignorance, fear and misconceptions surrounding the spiritual dimension can be challenged and removed only by having education and insight. Without education, nurses will not be able to provide positive and effective spiritual support to patients like those presented in this book. Nursing cannot boast of having a holistic approach until it starts to address the omissions that exist in relation to the spiritual dimension. As long as nursing sweeps over these omissions and limitations, patients will continue to receive a standard of care that is fragmented and not holistic.

It was with these strong emotions and personal opinions that I decided to undertake research to investigate this very subjective, personal dimension of our existence. The results of this research and personal experience have been used to inform and compile this book.

York 2000

Wilfred McSherry

Acknowledgements

I would like to thank all those individuals who have supported and encouraged me in this project. A special thank you goes to Jeanette Thompson (Lecturer, Department of Health Studies, University of York) for her comments and constructive criticism and to Student Nurses Emma Sunderland (Cohort 9) and Rob Reed (Cohort 10) for commenting upon style and level of draft chapters from a student perspective. Special thanks are due to Professor Keith Cash for writing the foreword and for his guidance and support in all matters academic. A final thank you goes to my wife Mandy and children Stacey and Matthew, who have had to sacrifice much to allow me to complete this project.

1

Spiritual heritage of nursing

INTRODUCTION

A study of the historical development of nursing reveals that it has a deep and rich spiritual heritage. It could be argued that nursing within modern societies emerged out of the ethos of the Judeo–Christian principle of charity – caring for those who were less fortunate than oneself. This chapter explores nursing's historical heritage, in which spirituality and nursing have always been synonymous, whether or not there has been a conscious realization of this by contemporary nurse theorists. This chapter also introduces some of the growing debate surrounding the effect that technological and medical advancement may have upon the relationship between spirituality and nursing.

Activity 1.1

Before proceeding with this chapter spend several minutes reflecting upon images associated with the word 'nurse'. Write down any words, thoughts or ideas that come to mind. Pay particular attention to some of the images in general uses, for example 'angel of mercy', patience and kindness.

SYMBOLS AND SIGNS

Your reflections may have revealed several terms, phrases or images associated with nursing (Box 1.1). Some of these may be historical in origin, indicating specific virtues such as patience, kindness or selfless dedication, while others may be related to garments of clothing such as uniforms or hats (remnants of the nun's habit and wimple). Modern interpretations may represent comedy as seen on seaside postcards, or the archetypal matron personified by Hatty Jacques, or even an object of desire as represented in the 'Carry On' films by Barbara Windsor.

By examining both the historical and modern images of nursing it is evident that there has been a dramatic shift in how nurses are perceived and portrayed in western society. The historical image of nurses as being morally virtuous has been replaced by images of comedy marketed by the mass media, who present nurses as objects of desire and ridicule. It would appear that respect for the sacred and spiritual values inherent in nursing has decayed. A possible explanation for this may be found in how the spiritual heritage of nursing is being eroded and replaced by modern, secular, material values. It is suggested that there is a subconscious attempt by western society to distance nursing from its past association with formal religious values and principles. This approach seems very negative and perhaps not representative of all sections in society. It could be argued that the negative attitude towards nursing is being challenged by television programmes that seek to portray nurses in a more professional manner, for example *Casualty* on British television and *ER* across the Atlantic. The remainder of this chapter will address some of these issues in more detail.

Box 1.1   Historical and modern images associated with nursing

Historical
  Symbol of virtues, kindness, caring
  An angel of mercy
  Uniform – remnant of the nun's habit
  Selflessness, vocation
Modern
  Comedy – 'Carry On' films, postcards
  Barbara Windsor – object of desire, envy, lust
  Archetypal matron – control subordination to medical profession
  Financial remuneration – career for life

HISTORICAL AND MODERN DEVELOPMENTS

A review of the literature addressing the spiritual dimension reveals that nursing has a strong historical affiliation with religious and spiritual traditions (Ellis 1980, Brittain & Boozer 1987, Allen 1991). Indeed, Smart (1969 p. 10) argues that to understand the developments of any society one must first gain insight into the religions that are found within it:

To understand human history and human life it is necessary to understand religion, and in the contemporary world one must understand other nations' ideologies and faith in order to grasp the meaning of life as seen from perspectives often very different from our own.

Therefore when exploring the spiritual heritage of nursing there is a fundamental need to become aware of the religious influences that have shaped and guided nursing throughout history. The outcome of Activity 1.1 reveals that nursing does have a strong formal religious and spiritual legacy that has influenced both the individual's and society's perceptions of nursing. The activity also indicates that those secular values and interpretations are replacing this rich spiritual heritage.

The strong association between mind, body, and spirit or soul was recognized by ancient civilizations. An imbalance in the spirit was believed to manifest itself through physical illness, disease, demonic possession or madness. During the Middle Ages people in western countries perceived the outbreak of disease or the presence of an illness as a punishment from God. People's experience of the physical, material world was intimately linked with the awareness of a higher power that controlled the individual's internal and external world, maintaining equilibrium and restoring order when chaos prevailed.

Tripartite being

Robbins (1991) suggests that the human is a tripartite being composed of mind, body and spirit. Although this illustration is divisive in that it fragments the individual, the analogy does indicate that the spiritual element must be in harmony with the physical and mental for spiritual development to occur. This realization of the importance of the spiritual dimension is reinforced in many religious teachings. It is not possible to provide an insight into the teachings of all world religions; here a brief overview of the Judeo–Christian approach is offered.

Awareness of a higher power

In the Old Testament the people of Israel awaited deliverance from their suffering and oppression. While in exile and journeying to the Promised Land their God rescued and delivered them from the hands of their captors. A higher authority had intervened in the destiny of humankind, restoring order and providing a template or code of living that governed and guided the beliefs, values and behaviours of the Jewish people.

This awareness of a higher power or divine being intervening in creation and controlling environmental, social, and individual destiny was not just specific to the Judeo–Christian tradition. Historically people have worshipped or offered sacrifices to the elements, fire, rain, sun and beasts in an attempt to improve their prosperity, indeed their chance of survival. Cupitt (1995 p. 90) writes:

The god may previously have been a tribal totem or clan divinity in animal form or a fertility figure . . .

The realization that a higher authority may control the destiny of humankind resulted in the emergence of different religions and cultures, all with their own forms of expression, beliefs, rituals and guiding principles.

Carson (1989) suggests that nursing has been steeped and fashioned by Christianity, a view shared by Ellis (1980 p. 42):

Did not nursing historically develop in a religious milieu in which love of God and mankind was expressed through care, compassion, and charity, to the sick, the poor, the orphans and the outcasts.

If one examines Ellis's quotation, then implicit within it is the notion of the Christian Beatitudes. It would appear that nursing in western society has been profoundly influenced by the teachings of Jesus Christ, whose values have shaped and guided many societies.

Carson (1989) presents an historical overview of the development of nursing. She describes one of the most famous of the religious orders, The Knights of Hospitallers of St John, who were responsible for establishing nursing and drew their members from crusaders, monks and religious brothers. This order was founded in the Middle Ages to provide nursing care for the victims of the crusades. Originally the order was located in Jerusalem but the congregation soon spread throughout the western world, providing nursing and spiritual care for the sick, and dying.

Modernism and secularism

From the argument presented so far you have probably deduced that we are living in an age that is dominated by things that are material and tangible, and where individuals want immediate results and rewards. Watson (1996 p. 39), recognizing the erosion of the spiritual dimension from the heart of nursing, writes:

May this era between centuries be the turning-point whereby nursing restores and further develops its caring–healing art and spiritual dimensions lest the profession collectively dies of a broken heart.

Watson warns that the spiritual dimension is the most important dimension of nursing in that it provides life to all other aspects of the profession. If nursing fails to restore the spiritual dimension to its central position, then nursing is in danger of being replaced by something dehumanizing and cold. Within the nursing literature the terms 'modernism' and 'secularism' are used with growing regularity. However, what do these words mean? And what are the implications of them upon the spiritual dimension of nursing?

If we focus upon our own existence and the things that are important to us, it is apparent that there are certain material things in life that are needed for survival such as food, shelter, warmth and water. Deprived of these important elements, we would die. Therefore by our very physical nature we are dependent upon material things. When the words modernism, materialistic and secular are used in nursing they are often used negatively to suggest that there is a preoccupation with or over-reliance upon them at the expense of other aspects such as the spiritual dimension. Narayanasamy (1997) proposes that the spiritual aspects of individuals will receive less attention in societies that are preoccupied with technological and scientific advancements and where individuals want immediate result or reward.

> **1.2** The three main 'isms'
>
> **Modernism**
>   The term used to describe an over-preoccupation with
>   modern technological, medical, scientific advancement
> **Secularism**
>   The belief that religious, spiritual principles have been made
>   redundant within modern cultures
> **Materialism**
>   An over-reliance with material objects and possessions at the
>   expense of recognizing the transcendent, mysterious aspects of
>   human existence

Modernism, materialism and secularism are the three main 'isms' that, in their extreme, seem to be incompatible with the notion of spirituality (Box 1.2). It is the emergence and subsequent preoccupation with these terms within nursing that has resulted in the demise of the spiritual heritage. An aditional form of extremism is the notion and misconception that spirituality equates only with formal, institutional religion, to which many individuals attach little importance (Burnard 1988, Narayanasamy 1991).

Scientific and technological advancement

If one thinks of the recent development within health care, in particular medical and surgical practices, then one cannot be surprised that these developments and innovations have changed the way in which society perceives health care. These changes are summed up by Donley (1991 p. 178):

Today, people expect that their diseased organs will be replaced and that disability and death will be postponed.

The innovations in scientific and medical technology mean nursing has become more complex and complicated. It would appear that the art and science of 'medicalization' dominate and guide practice while the spiritual dimension has been relegated from the premiere league to the second division. Science appears to be the predominant force guiding practice and shaping the direction and future of nursing. Bradshaw (1996a p. 61) alerts the scientific community to the hidden dangers in following this path:

It is not surprising that there should be a distrust of science as dehumanising and impersonal, mechanical, hard and cold. And certainly among nursing writers today, it is easy to trace a distrust with western science and what is called the biomedical.

Activity 1.2

Read the above quotation several times and see if you can think of any of your own examples from practice that may support the points that Bradshaw is making.

When reflecting upon the quotation it is easy to identify and recall examples from your own practice that confirm Bradshaw's apprehensions. How often does one still hear the phrase 'The appendicectomy in bed three', or more recently 'The lap chole (laparoscopic cholecystectomy) in bed four', the 'CABPG (coronary artery bypass graft) in bed five' or the 'CVA (cerebrovascular accident) in bed six', depending upon the specialty? This attitude towards individuals reflects the cold, dehumanizing face of science and a medical model that is not holistic, individualized or patient-centred.

Kearney (1994) and Bradshaw (1996a) suggest that science, religion and the spiritual realm are all seeking answers concerning the nature and mystery of our everyday life. Therefore, science and spirituality, instead of being in opposition, should be seen as different sides of the same coin that are closely united in seeking to find out the truths about our very existence and human condition. It is suggested that divisions arise because science and spirituality use different methods of enquiry to find out about the nature and structure of individuals. Science seeks to clarify by rigid control, producing evidence from experiments and trials, while spirituality is concerned with the 'touchy feely' aspects of our being that are often very mysterious and hard to pin down. It would appear the argument that there is no place for spirituality within the scientific community is redundant, short-sighted and misguided, since spirituality and science can work in harmony answering questions about our physical and existential world.

DEMISE OF SPIRITUALITY

It has been suggested that there has been a gradual demise of the spiritual dimension in the last years of the twentieth century. It has been suggested that the traditional view of nursing in which spirituality was fundamental have been replaced by a modern – 'fashionable' approach. Bradshaw (1993 p. 3) writes:

The long held Judeo–Christian, ethical tradition of caring for the sick as an altruistic calling was now seen as archaic, irrelevant and even a dangerous myth that needed dispelling – the opiate of oppressed nurses.

Bradshaw implies that many of nursing's historical and spiritual traditions have changed with advances in science and medicine. These changes contradict what several prominent twentieth century nurse theorists have written about holism and individualism (Peplau 1952, Henderson 1966, Orem 1985). Tournier (1954) suggested that there is a need for physicians to focus their interventions and treatments upon the patient rather than just the illness. Tournier (1954 p. 13) writes:

We may say, then, that every illness calls for two diagnoses: one scientific, nosological and causal, and the other spiritual, a diagnosis of its meaning and purpose.

Tournier had identified the need to treat both sides of the coin (scientific and spiritual), identifying and advocating holistic care. This position was quite unprecedented in that a physician had recognized how the scientific and the spiritual could be used to manage and treat the 'whole person' (Tournier 1973).

Activity 1.3

Spend some time reflecting upon what has been presented in the chapter so far. Make a list of possible explanations why many of nursing's traditional values have been replaced.

In the course of your reflection you may have identified several important reasons why the traditional values within nursing have been replaced. Some of these reasons may be associated with issues already discussed such as scientific and technological advancement, while others may be associated with changes in the way society views spirituality.

Dawson (1945) argued that since the Renaissance, a time of enlightenment, scientific growth and discovery of the natural world, western cultures have abandoned their religious heritage. Dawson (1945 p. 249) writes:

We have come to take it for granted that the unifying force in society is material interest, and that spiritual conviction is a source of strife and division. Modern civilization has pushed religion and the spiritual elements in culture out of the main stream of its development, so that they have lost touch with life and have become sectarianized and impoverished.

Dawson suggests that society's preoccupation with the temporal pervaded the philosophies of the medical profession and, more recently, nursing. Already in this chapter the dangers associated with the medical and surgical advances have been presented. The twentieth century has seen the development and rapid institution of the medical model (Swaffield 1988).

Female subordination

Another possible reason for the erosion of the spiritual heritage of nursing may be found in the authority and position that women held in society. It could be argued that nursing was inadvertently led into adopting a divisive medical model that sought to exclude the spiritual dimension because females in the earlier part of the twentieth century had little power. Swaffield (1988 p. 30) suggests that in the nursing and medical professions this resulted in female subordination. She states:

In caring for the sick, the nurse was to be trained to obey the orders of the doctor in an informed, but subordinate way. . . . It was impossible to develop such a system if there was any higher authority than the male doctor.

This subordination meant that the medical profession was at liberty to develop from a strictly scientific position, which may have led to the demise of the spiritual and religious values once present in nursing. The results of such developments signalled the end of many religious nursing orders. In this sense nursing became less of a vocation, and hospital managers took over the day-to-day control of these institutions.

However, recent announcements signal a possible change in the power relationships within health care. The UK Prime Minister Tony Blair has shown concern to reward the expertise of some nurse practitioners by creating a new 'consultant nurse'. These possible developments suggest that the medical profession no longer has a monopoly on patient care and that nurses have expert knowledge and skills to contribute to the ensuing debates concerning health care in the new millennium.

Advances in technology

Activity 1.4

Spend several minutes reflecting upon the technological advancements that have been introduced within health care.

Your reflections may have indicated that health care and nursing have witnessed the introduction of numerous technological advancements such as digital thermometers, infusion pumps and care-planning software. We are living in the age of technology. Almost every aspect of patient care can be measured or recorded electronically – the microchip and the computer dominate. It would appear that many tasks once performed by nurses are now no longer required (Harrison 1993). One cannot fail to see the advantages that technology has brought to patient care and the benefits of such innovations for the nurse in terms of effectiveness and efficiency in care delivery. However, the greatest hidden danger is that preoccupation with the technological aspects of care may prevent nurses from thinking or attending to the spiritual needs of patients. A computer, however effective in measuring blood pressure or central venous pressure, will be unable to communicate the warmth, affection, and sense of care that a single smile can transmit to a patient who may be feeling isolated or alone after admission. The inherent result of a preoccupation with technology is we fail to see the patient as an individual in the jurisdiction of our care.

Burkhardt and Nagai-Jacobson (1994 p. 19) share this concern. They write:

Increasing technology and the multiple pressures of busy clinics and hospitals are among forces that tend to focus efforts on nursing the equipment or treating diagnostic tests. In such times and settings, it is important that nurses remain cognizant of the value of maintaining caring connections with persons undergoing treatments and tests.

Vocation

When tracing the historical heritage of spirituality the notion of vocation is evident. Individuals in the past entered the nursing profession demonstrating the virtues of selflessness and sacrifice to care for those less fortunate. Bradshaw (1996 p. 42) shares this view when she writes:

. . . for it is clear that throughout history nursing was founded on an ethic and practice of spiritual care embodied in the nurse's vocation.

It is suggested that today many nurses, myself included, may be motivated by economic and capital gain while working in a profession that is saturated in the traditional value of selflessness (Swaffield 1988). Yet one cannot make judgements since we all need money and security of employment. Indeed, these are often quoted as being fundamental to an individual's spirituality in that they provide meaning, purpose and fulfilment. Therefore the reasons why individuals enter the nursing profession have changed. This may have an indirect effect on the erosion of some of the spiritual values once associated with the notion of vocation. It is not uncommon now when asking individuals their reasons for entering nursing to find that stability of career or a stepping stone to a better career are offered. Yet one cannot escape the fact that nursing takes a great deal from the individual's emotional and spiritual reserves even if one does not see nursing as a vocation.

Medicalization

One cannot explore the spiritual heritage of nursing and its subsequent decline without first examining the notion of medicalization. Some of the points previously discussed are related directly and indirectly to the concept. Medicalization within this section is taken to be a preoccupation with the developments in medical practice at the expense of other aspects of individuals that medicine seeks to serve. McCavery (1985 p. 129) draws attention to one of the main dangers associated with medicalization:

Today, secularization has permeated institutional care and has resulted in the designation of a low priority to all spiritual matters . . . The result has been an intense interest in the intricacies of medical science and unfortunately, a tendency to accord priority to the disease rather than a person.

As we have previously discussed, within health care the condition that was being treated seemed to be afforded more recognition than the individual that it affected or afflicted. A major concern with medicalization (medical/biological model) is its reductionist or systems-orientated approach, which sees individuals as a disease, for example a diabetic or an epileptic. Each of these conditions would be addressed within its own specialty, in the case of diabetes by an endocrinologist, while a neurologist would manage the epilepsy.

Another concern with medicalization is the misguided view that 'medicine knows best'. If individuals do not conform to expectations, for example a Jehovah's Witness refuses a blood transfusion, then he or she may be labelled as not conforming and having a disregard for medical opinion that could save his or her life. This point is explored in Case study 1.1.

Medicalization assumes that medicine knows what is best for all individuals who require treatment or are in need of health care. This case study suggests that if the woman had consented to the blood transfusion the outcome might have been

---

Case study 1.1 Who knows best?

A young woman is brought into the Accident and Emergency department with a massive gastrointestinal bleed presumed to be oesophageal varices. Immediately the medical and nursing teams start to resuscitate the woman and the consultant asks for 4 units of blood to be transfused. However, the woman interrupts and states that she does not want the blood transfusion because of her personal beliefs. Therefore other volume-expanding agents have to be used.
Unfortunately the woman dies from the haemorrhage several hours later. Talk around the department is, 'if only the woman had not refused a blood transfusion'. Others say, 'what a waste of life'. Yet the woman's husband says, 'God's will was done and she approached death as she believed was right'.

different. A positive aspect is that the medical management did abide by the woman's request for no blood – however, retrospectively the feeling was one of loss, sadness and regret – 'if only'. There seems to be a lack of sensitivity here, as individuals are making personal judgements and allowing their own prejudices towards different religious beliefs to influence their opinions towards the situation. This reaction is not uncommon, as Sampson (1982 p. 9) indicates:

Racial, cultural and religious matters can arouse strong personal feelings and distastes which may have a psychological or physical basis, and the hospital community is not immune to them.

Reappraisal of the case study should see individual staff pleased that the woman approached her death with dignity and she was supported positively in her own personal beliefs and values. This approach seems to be in conflict with medicalization that is concerned at all costs with preserving life and health. It would seem that medicalization and spirituality are incompatible.

The medical model does not look at individuals holistically in that all aspects of a person are interconnected. A physician will look at all the signs and symptoms and the results of investigations to arrive at a diagnosis to treat the system that is diseased or affected. A problem arises when the disease itself is caused by something not physical but psychological, social or spiritual in origin. For example, an elderly lady refuses to eat or drink because she has been taken into residential care and her home sold to pay for her care costs. A nutritional assessment will reveal malnutrition and her urea and electrolytes (U & E) profile will indicate dehydration. The physician may treat both these factors. However, the fundamental issue of her loss of meaning and purpose in life may be neglected if only the medical model is used.

Medicalization of patient care needs to be considered against the individual's own personal beliefs and values. Sampson (1982) highlights a possible solution to the problems linked with medicalization. One suggestion is the development of cultural awareness and sensitivity. Each new medical or surgical development may have different implication upon patients' personal values or religious beliefs. An example of this may be asking a woman who is having a hysterectomy how she may feel about having to have her ovaries removed and commencing on hormone replacement therapy if this is found to be necessary during the operation. By generating awareness into all aspects of an individual's life information will be elicited that will enable health care to be provided that will satisfy and take into consideration personal beliefs and values. This approach will go some way to remove the assumption of 'we know what's best' that has been equated with medicalization.

REVERSAL IN OPINION

It has been suggested that the spiritual dimension of nursing has been eroded and replaced by more secular and modern views. Modernism, secularism and materialism seem to be the guiding forces in health care. Colliton (1981) and Clark et al (1991) indicate that there is a change in opinion, a revitalization and a universal recognition of the importance of refocusing upon patients holistically, paying particular attention to the spiritual dimension. Bradshaw (1994, p. 332) writes:

The lamp has been shattered. To its surprise nursing finds itself today in the dark, and no matter how it tries to integrate the many different fragments of glass, it cannot achieve the organic unity of care.

Bradshaw highlights the consequences that the erosion of nursing's spiritual heritage has had upon the profession. It would appear that nursing is in the dark, seeking direction and a new meaning for its diverse roles and responsibilities.

 Activity 1.5

Can you think of any legislation that suggests that nurses should be attending to the spiritual needs of their patients?

National

Within the UK there is an attempt to rediscover and focus upon the spiritual dimension within the health care settings. Your reflection may have identified several pieces of national and statutory legislation that currently guide nursing practice. The need to focus upon spiritual and cultural issues has been recognized by the Government, which published the Patient's Charter. The Patient's Charter (HMSO 1992) presents nine Standards. The first Standard deals with issues concerning spirituality:

... respect for privacy, dignity and religious and cultural beliefs.

The word spirituality is not explicitly used in the Standard but is implied since the issues addressed within this Standard pertain to fundamental areas surrounding the spiritual dimension.

Professional

The importance of spirituality has not only been recognized nationally, but also professionally. The United Kingdom Central Council for Nursing Midwifery and Health Visiting, which governs and guides professional practice, alludes to the spiritual dimension in its Professional Code of Conduct (UKCC 1992). The code encourages nurses to address any limitations in their practice knowledge that may be detrimental to the patients' or clients' interests. Clause seven suggests that nurses should recognize and respect the uniqueness of individuals irrespective of religious and cultural beliefs. Again, inferences can be made from this clause and applied to spirituality, which is often shaped by culture, or an individual's own unique belief and value system. Therefore if spirituality is inadequately addressed, then nurses are only partially adhering to the code.

Statutory

A third piece of statutory guidance that you might be aware of is the practice competency statements issued by the National Boards for Nursing. The late 1980s saw the implementation of *Project 2000 – A New Preparation for Practice* (UKCC 1986), which lists competencies every student ought to achieve, irrespective of branch, for registration on the national register. Competency xiv (p. 41) reads:

Identify physical, psychological, social, and spiritual needs of the patient or client; be aware of and value the concept of individual care, devise a plan of care, contribute to its implementation and evaluation by demonstrating an appreciation and practice of the problems solving approach.

This quotation highlights the growing realization by the nursing profession that care provided should be holistic and individualized. This position is a shift or reversal of that which operates around the biological or medical model discussed above. The quotation underlines the responsibility that educational institutions have in providing student nurses with the necessary skills in order to address and meet patients' spiritual needs in practice. Issues surrounding spirituality and education are explored in greater detail in Chapter 7.

Growing awareness

A search of any of the databases currently available in any university library addressing the subject of spirituality in nursing would reveal that a steady flow of articles has been published since the 1950s. However, in the UK this interest with the spiritual dimension has only gained momentum since the late 1980s. This refocusing upon the spiritual dimension supports the views presented in this chapter that the importance of addressing a patient's spiritual needs is crucial to that individual's health and sense of well-being, something which science and medicine cannot do alone (Thompson 1984).

Within the UK there are annual conferences and interest groups addressing the subject of spirituality and several books (at different levels) have been published. Management's attention has been drawn to the need to assess and evaluate the effectiveness of care provision in this area. To this end a framework for the provision of spiritual care has been devised (Institute of Nursing 1995, Keighley 1997). These innovations reinforce the attempts by nurse theorists, educators and researchers to place the spiritual dimension firmly on the health care agenda, putting spirituality at the centre of health care. This growing public awareness of the importance of spirituality for an individual's sense of well-being and quality of life has helped to dispel and remove many of the misconceptions that have shrouded spirituality and its place within nursing (Ross 1995).

The increasing amounts of different types of literature and research being published generate new and deeper insights into the spiritual dimension. It is suggested that a new more universal approach and acceptance of the spiritual dimension is emerging that is challenging all health care professions to evaluate their own attitudes and perceptions towards this fundamental aspect of individualized care. As we enter the new millennium it would appear that the technological age is passing, being replaced with recognition of the need to return and reinvest in the caring and spiritual heritage of nursing. We are now entering the age of spirituality and spiritual enlightenment. All health care professions and all those involved in the provision of patient care need to capitalize and contribute towards this growing debate so that the most efficient and effective care can be developed. Keighley (1997 p. 51) in concluding his article addressing the 'Organisational structures and personal spiritual belief' writes:

Whatever the stimulus, it is clear that there is an opportunity to rethink approaches and structures. If this is achieved in an integrated way, then the benefits to care receivers and caregivers could be very significant indeed.

CONCLUSION

This chapter traced briefly and superficially some of the historical and modern developments that surround the spiritual heritage of nursing. The arguments and evidence presented suggest that the debates concerning the erosion of nursing's spiritual heritage and the notion of medicalization are complex and diverse. The emergence of the three 'isms', modernism, secularism and materialism, indicate that society has lost awareness of things sacred and spiritual. Preoccupation with the technological and material have replaced the notion of holistic and individualized care, at the centre of which rests spirituality. However it is argued that there is now a reawakening of interest in the spiritual dimension in maintaining an individual's health and sense of well-being. This refocusing upon the spiritual dimension has seen health care, and indeed society, enter a new era of spiritual enlightenment.

REFERENCES

Allen C 1991 The inner light. Nursing Standard 5 (20): 52–53
Bradshaw A 1993 Lighting the lamp: the covenant as an encompassing
   framework for the spiritual dimension of nursing care. In: Farmer E (ed.) 1996
   Exploring the spiritual dimension of care. Quay Books, Lancaster

Bradshaw A 1994 Lighting the lamp: the spiritual dimension of nursing care. Scutari Press, London

Bradshaw A 1996 The legacy of Nightingale. Nursing Times 92 (6): 42–43

Bradshaw A 1996a Does science need religion? In: Farmer E (ed.) Exploring the spiritual dimension of care. Quay Books, Lancaster

Brittain J N, Boozer J 1987 Spiritual care: integration into a collegiate nursing curriculum. Journal of Nurse Education 26 (4): 155–160

Burkhardt M A, Nagai-Jacobson M G 1994 Reawakening spirit in clinical practice. Journal of Holistic Nursing 12 (1): 9–21

Burnard P 1988 The spiritual needs of atheists and agnostics. Professional Nurse (December): 130–132

Carson V B 1989 Spiritual dimensions of nursing practice. W B Saunders, Philadelphia

Clark C C, Cross J R, Deane D M, Lowry L W 1991 Spirituality integral to quality care. Holistic Nursing Practice 5 (3): 67–76

Colliton M A 1981 The spiritual dimension of nursing. In: Beland I L, Passos J Y (eds) Clinical Nursing, 4th edn. Macmillan, New York

Cuppitt D 1997 After God: the future of religion. Weidenfeld & Nicolson, London

Dawson C 1945 Progress and religion: an historical enquiry. Sheed and Ward, London

Donley R 1991 Spiritual dimensions of health care nursing's mission. Nursing and Health Care 12 (4): 178–183

Ellis D 1980 Whatever happened to the spiritual dimension? The Canadian Nurse 76 (8): 42–43

Harrison J 1993 Spirituality and nursing practice. Journal of Clinical Nursing 2: 211–217

Henderson V 1966 Nature of nursing. Macmillan, New York

HMSO 1992 The patient's charter. HMSO, London

Hubert S M 1963 Spiritual care for every patient. Journal of Nurse Education 2 (6): 9–11

Institute of Nursing 1995 A framework for spiritual, faith and related pastoral care. Institute of Nursing, University of Leeds, Leeds

Kearney S 1994 Spirituality as a coping mechanism in multiple sclerosis: the patient's perspective. Unpublished BSc dissertation, Institute of Nursing Studies, University of Hull, Hull

Keighley T 1997 Organisational structures and personal spiritual belief. International Journal of Palliative Nursing 3 (1): 47–51

McCavery R 1985 Spiritual care in acute illness. In: McGilloway P, Myco F (eds) Nursing and spiritual care. Harper & Row, London

Narayanasamy A 1991 Spiritual care: a resource guide. Quay Books, Lancaster

Narayanasamy A 1997 Spiritual dimensions of learning disability. In: Gates B, Beacock C (eds) Dimensions of learning disability. Baillière Tindall, London

Orem D E 1985 Nursing: concepts of practice, 3rd edn. McGraw-Hill, New York

Peplau H E 1952 Interpersonal relations in nursing. G P Putnam & Sons, New York

Robbins C 1991 Spiritual care in a multi-cultural society. Pacemaker (October): 1–3

Ross L 1995 The spiritual dimension: its importance to patients' health, well-being and quality of life and its implications for nursing practice. International Journal of Nursing Studies 32 (5): 457–468

Sampson C 1982 The neglected ethic: religious and cultural factors in the care of patients. McGraw-Hill, London

Smart N 1969 The religious experience of mankind. Collins, London

Swaffield L 1988 Religious roots. Nursing Times 84: 28–30
Thompson J H 1984 Spiritual considerations in the prevention, treatment and
cure of disease. Oriel Press, London
Tournier P 1954 A doctor's case book in the light of the Bible. SCM Press,
London
Tournier P 1973 Paul Tournier's medicine of the whole person. Word Books,
Waco, Texas
UKCC 1986 Project 2000 – A new preparation for practice. UKCC, London
UKCC 1992 The code of professional conduct. UKCC, London
Watson J 1996 Art, caring, spirituality and humanity. In: Farmer E (ed.)
Exploring the spiritual dimension of care. Quay Books, Lancaster

FURTHER READING

*This selection of literature will develop your understanding and insight into the
complex debates surrounding nursing's spiritual heritage. These texts will
provide a richer and deeper insight into the religious organizations that have
shaped and guided nursing's spiritual heritage. Sampson's work in particular is
a seminal piece of work addressing religious and cultural factors associated
with patient care. Despite being a little dated, this book still has a great deal
to offer.*

Bradshaw A 1996 Does science need religion? In: Farmer E (ed.) Exploring the
spiritual dimension of care. Quay Books, Lancaster
Carson V B 1989 Spiritual dimensions of nursing practice. W B Saunders,
Philadelphia, section 2
Keighley T 1997 Organisational structures and personal spiritual belief.
International Journal of Palliative Nursing 3 (1): 47–51
McCavery R 1985 Spiritual care in acute illness In: McGilloway P, Myco F (eds)
Nursing and spiritual care. Harper & Row, London
Robbins C 1991 Spiritual care in a multi-cultural society. Pacemaker (October):
1–3
Sampson C 1982 The neglected ethic: religious and cultural factors in the care
of patients. McGraw-Hill, London
Swaffield L 1988 Religious roots. Nursing Times 84: 28–30

2

Spirituality explored

INTRODUCTION

This chapter explores the concept of spirituality and explains why it is difficult to define. The chapter demonstrates that spirituality is individually determined and often finds expression and meaning in the ordinary and mundane aspects of life. Definitions of spirituality are presented and discussed within the context of nursing. The key terms spiritual need and spiritual well-being, which are used in connection with the spiritual dimension, are introduced.

MAKING SENSE

The need to understand and investigate the elusive concept of spirituality has generated much interest and debate within the nursing profession (Simsen 1985, Waugh 1992, Harrison 1993, Bradshaw 1994, Wright 1997, McSherry 1998). This chapter presents and explores aspects of the spiritual dimension that assist in defining and making sense of the concept in relation to nursing. However, a major question arises as to how one can begin to approach and 'make sense' of such diverse, abstract and subjective aspects of holistic nursing practice.

Several authors (Stoll 1989, Narayanasamy 1991, Harrison 1993, McSherry 1997) have explored and identified an inventory of elements that are categorized under the 'umbrella' term of spirituality. These include spiritual needs, spiritual distress, spiritual well-being and a general analysis of the words spirit and spirituality. It would appear that all these terms are interrelated. An investigation into each approach reveals and 'sheds light' on different facets of this multidimensional and mysterious aspect of life.

THE LIVED EXPERIENCE

One way of learning to understand what is meant by the term spirituality is by reflecting upon what the term means to ourselves.

Activity 2.1

Before reading the rest of this chapter, spend a few moments reflecting upon the word spirituality. Write down the thoughts, feelings and images that come to mind while reflecting upon its meaning.

Having undertaken Activity 2.1 you will now appreciate that spirituality is often something that we may not consciously think about and when asked to describe spirituality we may find it difficult to articulate either a definition or a description. In describing spirituality you may have jotted down several points:

some pertaining to religion such as a belief in a God or a Supreme Being

more general terms surrounding life such as relationships, beliefs, values, ideologies

or even issues surrounding death and belief in an after life.

This reflection leads on to Activity 2.2.

Activity 2.2

Having thought about what the word spirituality means to you, now consider and reflect upon the things in life that you most value, e.g. family, friends, health, and anything that is important to you as an individual.

Having thought about the word spirituality and reflected upon the things we value, one starts to appreciate why spirituality is something that we may take for granted. We all have an awareness and sense of importance towards certain things in life (revealed in Activity 2.2) that are personal and unique. By reflecting upon these things it becomes apparent that everyday rituals, practices and people provide us with much of life's meaning, purpose and fulfilment. However, we may never attach any spiritual significance to them. By spending several moments thinking about the things in life that we value, one can soon produce a list of items, for example, health, family, friends, career, etc., that are fundamental to our existence and being. An analysis of this list reveals that many of the things that we take for granted link in with the concept of spirituality in that these are aspects of life that generate much of life's meaning, purpose and fulfilment. If we are deprived of any of these because of illness, loss, or misfortune life can soon lose meaning and we can find ourselves questioning our existence at a very deep level, searching for answers and solutions. These important issues will be explored and discussed in a little more depth below in the section 'The ordinary and mundane'.

Having reflected upon the word spirituality several important themes begin to emerge. The word spirituality may be interpreted differently by individuals. There is a uniqueness and originality in the way that we perceive the concept. However, what does become evident is that there are certain elements of the subject that are universal and applicable to us all. Spirituality does not only apply to the religious person but to every individual irrespective of religious affiliation. Emerging from this universality is the need for sensitivity when discussing this very personal concept.

Caution

Caution must be used when attempting to define the concept of spirituality, as there is a need for sensitivity. This approach is required since spirituality is a mysterious and complex dimension of our being and existence. It is mysterious in that spirituality involves aspects of daily life that are deeply personal and sensitive such as religion and religious affiliation, and complex in that it involves aspects of life that are intimately interwoven into the tapestry of beliefs, values and cultures. These are all aspects of life that individuals may find it hard to discuss, define and talk about openly (think back to Activity 2.1 – did you find it difficult?). In conclusion, the individual interprets spirituality differently. This interpretation will be influenced by personal identity and life experiences. This must be borne in mind when trying to define spirituality because there is always the danger of applying our own definitions of spirituality to others. This can only be avoided if we are sensitive and understand the personal nature of spirituality in a non-judgemental way.

ASSOCIATED TERMS

To broaden and expand our understanding of the subject of spirituality we need to explore other important aspects and terms that make up the spiritual dimension, mentioned earlier in this chapter. Figure 2.1 shows how all the terms associated

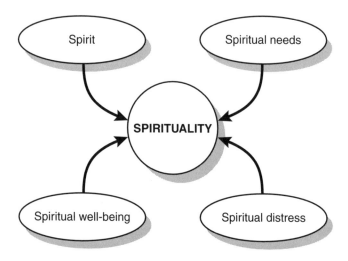

Figure 2.1 Terms associated with definitions of spirituality.

with spirituality or the spiritual dimension are interrelated and connected. Each term will be addressed in detail throughout the rest of this chapter.

THE HUMAN SPIRIT DEFINED

Origins of the word

The word 'spirit' has its origins from the Latin word *spiritus*, which generates images of life, breath, wind and air. The word 'spirit' relates to the unique spirit of an individual that is their life force, the essence and energy of their being. It is this force that develops in an individual the ability to transcend the natural laws and orders of this life, allowing access to a mysterious or transcendent dimension. The 'spirit' drives and motivates individuals to find meaning and purpose, allowing expression in all aspects and experiences of life, especially in times of crisis and need.

Meanings associated with the word

Several authors (Dickinson 1975, Shelly & Fish 1988, Stoll 1989) have investigated the concept of spirituality by first exploring possible meanings associated with the word 'spirit'. Everyday usage of the word is illustrated by the definition in *The Oxford Paperback Dictionary*, which provides numerous descriptions of the word, the majority of which may help to demystify the use of the word:

1. a person's mind or feelings or animating principle as distinct from his body, *shall be with you in spirit.* 2. soul. 3. a disembodied soul, a ghost. 4. life and consciousness not associated with a body, *God is pure spirit; the Spirit,* the Holy Spirit (see holy). 5. a person's nature. 6. a person with certain mental or moral qualities, *a few brave spirits went swimming.* 7. the characteristic quality or mood of something, *the spirit of the times; the spirit of the law,* its real purpose as distinct from a strict interpretation of its word.

The above definitions suggest that the 'spirit' of a person is an entity on its own. They also suggest that it is an animating life force present within all individuals. It is also described as a frame of mind or attitude towards life.

Stoll (1989) describes a person's spirit as the *Imago dei* (Image of God) that is present within every person, making him or her a thinking, feeling, moral, creative being able to relate meaningfully to God (as defined by the person), self and others. Stoll is referring directly to the *Book of Genesis* (2: 7), which reads:

Yahweh God fashioned man of dust from the soil. Then he
breathed into his nostrils a breath of life, and thus man became a
living being.

This quotation infers that it is this 'breath of life' that distinguishes and separates humankind from the rest of the animal kingdom because individuals are made in the likeness of God, whose presence resides within them in a mystical union. This perspective is orientated and focused in the Judeo–Christian tradition. Yet even the Atheist and Agnostic still possess a spirit or attitude towards life (Burnard 1988). The suggestion of an animating force or principle is supported by Dickinson (1975 p. 1790), who states:

Spirit is the animating but intangible principle that gives liveliness to
the physical organism as well as the literal breath of life.

DEFINITIONS OF SPIRITUALITY

After exploring the word 'spirit', the next step is to try and define what is meant by the word 'spirituality'. It was stated earlier that the concept of spirituality is gaining much attention within the nursing press (Bradshaw 1996, McSherry 1996, Turner 1996, Wright 1997). A study of these articles soon reveals that the definitions presented are very descriptive, anecdotal and rhetorical, presenting the views and opinions of individuals, which cannot be generalized and applied to the general population. However, these articles do contribute to our understanding of the concept in that they provide us with an insight into what people feel and think about spirituality.

Among the numerous descriptive definitions of spirituality that are to be found in the literature, there are several that have been developed and used in research studies to provide a framework for investigation. One such definition of spirituality, which has been quoted and referred to in many texts, is that presented by Murray & Zentner (1989 p. 259). According to these authors, spirituality is:

A Quality that goes beyond religious affiliation, that strives for inspirations, reverence, awe, meaning and purpose, even in those who do not believe in any good. The spiritual dimension tries to be in harmony with the universe, and strives for answers about the infinite, and comes into focus when the person faces emotional stress, physical illness or death.

If we read this definition several times and reflect upon its meaning and significance to health care, particularly its relevance to nursing, several important themes may begin to emerge:

spirituality is a universal concept relevant to all individuals
the uniqueness of each individual is paramount
formal religious affiliation is not a prerequisite of spirituality
an individual may become more spiritually aware during a
   time of need.

This definition highlights the complex and subjective nature of spirituality, reinforcing the notion of mystery and transcendence. It demonstrates how all aspects of life – physical, psychological and social – are interrelated and interconnected. From this definition it would appear that spirituality is concerned with an individual's past, present and future, especially when facing illness or the prospect of death. Reed (1992 p. 350) adopts a similar description of spirituality when she writes:

Specifically spirituality refers to the propensity to make meaning through a sense of relatedness to dimensions that transcend the self in such a way that empowers and does not devalue the individual. This relatedness may be experienced intrapersonally (as a connectedness within oneself), interpersonally (in the context of others and the natural environment) and transpersonally (referring to a sense of relatedness to the unseen, God, or power greater than the self and ordinary source).

Reed's definition suggests that spirituality is concerned with the individual and his or her relationship with others and the environment, also reaffirming the notion that spirituality involves an awareness of something greater or beyond oneself (the mystical nature inherent in every individual).

Earlier you were asked (Activity 2.2) to reflect upon the things in life that bring you value and meaning. The two definitions of spirituality presented in this chapter suggest that it embrace all aspects of life that bring value and meaning, since they imply that spirituality is concerned with everyday events and concerns such as relationships, health, career, etc. Academics may argue that this is an oversimplification of the concept. However, if spirituality is to be relevant to nursing and applied in clinical practice, then spirituality must be defined in a manner that makes it both meaningful and relevant for patients and nurses.

The ordinary and mundane

During a workshop on spirituality one of the co-facilitators, a chaplain, made a useful observation concerning the word spirituality. Incorporated in the middle of the word spirituality is found the word 'ritual', a word well known by nurses (Walsh & Ford 1989). What has this point to do with spirituality? Ritual means a regulated or repeated action, and this can be applied to religious practices and ordinary aspects of life. Within the context of a religious ceremony prayers or actions are carried out according to historical customs and practices, for example the marriage ceremony. An example from nursing may be the ritual of recording daily observation without really asking if they are necessary. It would appear that all individuals require ritual and routine because it provides structure and security. Therefore if one applies these principles to spirituality it would seem that the word is concerned with ordinary events and routines of daily living. The definition offered by Murray & Zentner supports the idea that spirituality is concerned with the ordinary and mundane ritualistic events of life. This may appear a contradiction since the use of the word mundane implies an absence of the spiritual. However, if one reflects upon daily living it is often the mundane rituals such as going to work, doing the washing or walking the dog that bring meaning and purpose to everyday life. As suggested earlier, these ordinary and often mundane tasks are usually taken for granted, and the fulfilment derived from them is not recognized until an event occurs that causes a break in normal practices.

This is illustrated in Case study 2.1. John's situation highlights that it is the everyday tasks and rituals that give structure, meaning and purpose. Nurses will encounter numerous patients like John who are trying to find new meaning as their

> **Case study 2.1**
>
> John, aged 75, is admitted into hospital with a chest infection. While admitting John the nurse enquires about his occupation. He replies, 'I'm recently retired. I was a school teacher – and do you know something? I didn't think I'd miss it – all the hassle – when I retired, but I do! Life seems to have lost some of its meaning, now that I don't work.'

roles and lives change. It is important to recognize that spirituality is not just concerned with matters of theology and existential beliefs, but about the ordinary and the mundane.

One important point to consider when trying to establish a definition of spirituality is not to make the subject complex and produce a definition that may be authoritative. The way forward is to think of spirituality in terms of its relevance and importance to individuals in their everyday existence. All people irrespective of creed, culture, race or religion have a spirituality that is uniquely interpreted and determined by their everyday situation.

Spirituality does not only equal religion

In an article entitled 'The inner light', Allen (1991) suggests that nurses would be more scandalized to find a Bible in a patient's property bag than a copy of the *Karma Sutra*. Allen is highlighting the misconceptions surrounding spirituality and religion. In the past the word spirituality has been used synonymously with religion. Any mention of the word spirituality either implied that a patient required the services of the hospital chaplain or that a nurse who attended to such patients was in need of a psychiatric referral. If one adopts such a narrow definition of the word and applies it only to the religious and pious, then there is a danger that a large proportion of patients and indeed nurses may not have their spirituality needs addressed. For some individuals, patients and nurses, the religious aspect and the belief in a God will be fundamental and central to their interpretation of spirituality. However, if this definition were applied to all individuals it would be extremely inappropriate and possibly offensive. It appears that in today's society these two words are in conflict or opposition, the spiritual/religious versus the secular and materialistic. Yet this conflict only arises if one chooses to be judgemental in the interpretation of the word spirituality by adopting a narrow definition. Tolerance, understanding and flexibility have to be used and applied when defining spirituality. Only by being tolerant to each individual's religious orientation or political and philosophical persuasion will a true understanding of spirituality be gained. If one adopts this approach then these two words will not be viewed in opposition but as elements or threads that contribute and make up the larger tapestry of spirituality.

Analogy and symbolism

The word spirituality is perceived and used differently by all individuals. By adopting this individualist approach the meaning of the word becomes mysterious and subjective in that the term may mean different things to individuals within differing contexts. One way in which individuals, and indeed societies, try to describe or define the word is by using analogy and symbolism. An example can be found in the way that religions use drawings to illustrate their God(s). Ancient peoples drew figures of animals that they worshipped because they provided food. This approach can be applied to spirituality because images or illustrations with which people are familiar assist in providing visual stimulation and insight, allowing the hidden meanings or interpretations of the word to be revealed.

Mountain range

Life is depicted as a journey or pilgrimage. Sometimes the route and the scenes are beautiful and idyllic. Yet there are times when the mountains are steep and difficult to ascend, and no sooner does one conquer one peak than another appears on the horizon that is much higher and steeper. Life and spirituality is like this for most individuals. At one period in time a person may be experiencing hardship and conflict that may be manifested as illness, disease or bereavement (the steep slopes). Yet there are many occasions when a person experiences joy and happiness, life is running smoothly and calmly, and everything seems to fall into place with little effort (the scenic routes). This analogy suggests that life can be difficult and that at some point events may occur that confront, challenge and test us. It is during this journey that a person's spirituality is shaped and developed. This raises the notion that spirituality can be developed. In fact several authors have suggested that spirituality changes and evolves across a lifespan (Erikson 1963, Carson 1989). Our spirituality is not completed overnight, nor is it something static; rather it is transient and always in a state of flux. It is the spirit's ability to adjust and change to situations, either religious or secular, that will ultimately shape an individual's spirituality.

A football

The world cup and league football provide entertainment for many, and hopefully joy for the victorious. The football (Fig. 2.2) provides another analogy for spirituality (McSherry & Draper 1998). Here we consider that spirituality is made up of many component parts (patches) all stitched together to make the (ball) or person. The leather patches each represent a different aspect of spirituality. Each aspect is attached and interrelated to the next because they are stitched tightly together. All the patches share the same importance and cannot function in isolation. The football can be burst and/or punctured, requiring repair. This happens in both daily life and the spiritual life, when occasionally circumstances occur that knock the air out of us. These events are usually unexpected and beyond our control. Often the person is left asking the question 'why?', and searching for some meaning or purpose in the event. The football takes many kicks during the match – here the match represents the arena of life and the ball represents our spirituality or the individual.

SPIRITUAL NEEDS

As living functional, volitional and interactive creatures we have certain basic physiological, social and psychological needs that are fundamental to our survival, for example a physical

Activity 2.3

There exists within nursing a debate surrounding spiritual needs. What are they, and do we all have spiritual needs?

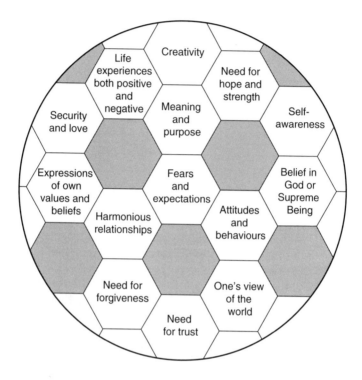

Figure 2.2 The analogy of spirituality as a football shows the complexity of the concept, involving many dimensions.

need for food and water (Dunn 1993). Deprived from these necessities for prolonged periods we soon dehydrate, starve and die.

Labun (1988) suggests that spirituality is expressed and shaped by the accepted practices and beliefs of a particular culture. This approach to spirituality implies that spiritual needs have their origin in the institutional religious domains, intimating at a belief in God or a deity. It appears that spiritual needs have an intrinsic and extrinsic value and meaning: their relevance and value to the individual is intrinsic, and their relationship with the universe at large is extrinsic. Stallwood & Stoll (1975 p. 1088) define spiritual needs as:

Any factors necessary to establish and maintain a person's dynamic personal relationship with God (as defined by that individual) . . . and out of that relationship to experience forgiveness . . ., love . . ., hope . . ., trust . . . meaning and purpose in life.

Stallwood & Stoll demonstrate that spiritual needs are not purely associated with religion or belief in God but a semantic philosophy towards life (a search for meaning and purpose). Colliton (1981) stresses that spiritual needs are a requirement that touches the core of one's being where the search for personal meaning takes place.

Victor Frankl (1987 p. 74), a survivor of the World War II concentration (extermination) camps and the founder of a Vienna School of Existential Psychotherapy, stresses people's search for meaning and purpose when he states:

The prisoner who had lost faith in the future – his future – was doomed. With his loss of belief in the future, he also lost his spiritual hold; he let himself decline and become subject to mental and physical decay.

Frankl goes on to say that meaning must be specific and have purpose to the individual. Travelbee (1966 p. vii) believes that:

A major belief is that human beings are motivated by a search for meaning in all life experiences, and meaning can be found in the experiences of illness, suffering and pain.

It is the nurse's role to assist individuals to make sense and find meaning in such times of crisis such as the acceptance of a terminal diagnosis, the loss of a loved one, or adapting to life with a permanent disability. These approaches presented by Frankl (1987) and Travelbee (1966) suggests that spiritual needs are seen as the deepest requirements of self. If an individual is able to identify and fulfil these requirements then he or she can function harmoniously, finding meaning, value, purpose and hope in life even when life may be threatened (Harrison 1993).

Several nurse authors (Highfield & Cason 1983, Shelly & Fish 1988, Narayanasamy 1991) have identified and categorized a litany of items that can be included in the classification of spiritual needs. Shelly & Fish (1988) identified three spiritual needs:

the need for meaning and purpose
the need for love and relatedness
the need for forgiveness.

It must be stressed that Shelly & Fish base their work upon a Judeo–Christian approach to spirituality. Therefore for the

Christian it is Jesus Christ who is identified as the main person able to satisfy all people's deepest yearnings and spiritual needs. Shelly & Fish suggest that nurses may be called upon to function in a pastoral role, in order that a patient's spiritual and religious needs are addressed during periods of hospitalization when a patient may be isolated or prevented from maintaining his or her own unique individual religious practices.

Highfield & Cason (1983) used a spiritual needs approach in their descriptive study investigating surgical nurses' awareness of spiritual concerns. The researchers identified four spiritual needs:

the need for meaning and purpose in life
the need to give and receive love
the need for hope
the need for creativity.

Interestingly, Highfield & Cason leave the definition or interpretation of God up to the individual's own perceptions and beliefs. The work of these authors broadens and widens the boundaries of spiritual needs. There is a shift away from the religious aspects of life to include other fundamental and valuable concepts – which are still spiritual in origin – although the main thrust focuses around meaning and purpose, fulfilment and value in life.

Narayanasamy (1991) highlights the inclusion of other spiritual needs by applying the concept directly to nursing care. Like the previous authors, he lists:

the need for meaning and purpose
the need for love and harmonious relationships
the need for forgiveness
the need for a source of hope and strength
creativity.

However, he identifies and lists a further four spiritual needs:

a need for trust
the need for expression of personal beliefs and values
the need for spiritual practices
expressions of God or deity.

These spiritual needs are explained in more detail in Box 2.1. They demonstrate that a spiritual need may originate from any facet of our human existence, whether it be physiological, psychological or sociological. It stresses the importance of an holistic approach to health care. There is a dynamic interplay and exchange of the spiritual dimension with all the other realms of our existence. The confusion arises when a spiritual need is viewed in isolation or when an individual is fragmentalized, thus obscuring the whole meaning. An individual may express a need for a harmonious relationship, after having experienced a marital breakdown. The more psychologically oriented may see this as a psychological need, when in reality the individual is expressing a desire to explore issues that are fundamental, unique and central to their existence – spiritual in nature, originating from the psychosocial dimensions. Likewise it would be a grave misconception and error to infer that an atheist or an agnostic does not have spiritual needs because they do not share a belief in a God or deity (Burnard 1988).

Box 2.1 Spiritual needs explained

Meaning and purpose
We all have a desire and need to identify some meaning in our lives and existence that will assist in generating motivation or purpose, which will lead to a sense of fulfilment. This search is undertaken in health and during times of illness.

Love and harmonious relationships
Without the intimacy and comfort gained by sharing with others, e.g. a spouse, partner or close friends, we can feel isolated, alone and deprived of touch, security and love. These are all important needs derived from personal contact and involvement with people. However, can the same love be generated or experienced by close contact with animals and creation?

Need for forgiveness
At times life can be troublesome and conflicts do emerge. However, unresolved anger, and guilt can lead to loss of physical, psychological, social and spiritual well-being. Therefore in order to maintain an equilibrium there is a need to try and resolve conflict in life and at times forgiveness is sought.

Need for a source of hope and strength
Spirituality is often referred to as a source of inner strength and hope. Personal beliefs, values and attitudes can bring hope in people, the future or from a religious perspective, such as life everlasting, enabling individuals to draw strength from their convictions and commitment.

Creativity
The ability to find meaning, expression and value in aspects of life such as literature, art, music and other activities, which originate from

the creative nature of individuals, provides expression and meaning as well as a means of communication. Creativity can be inspirational, elevating people's emotions and feelings to the beauty present in creation.

Trust
Individuals can become isolated and neglected when deprived of trust. Trust can be applied to the individual, family, friends or society – the world at large. Trust is a prerequisite for establishing friendships and therapeutic relationships. By adopting this approach it would appear that trust is fundamental to existence and communication. Trust leads to a sense of value, self-worth and acceptance by others.

Maintain spiritual practices
As we progress through life certain spiritual practices may be developed and fashioned. These practices may originate from within a religious framework, such as the need for daily prayer or attendance at church services or the synagogue. However an individual may have grown spiritually through a weekly walk in the countryside or by taking part in sports. During periods of illness or hospitalization there will be a need to ensure such practices are continued where possible.

Express one's own belief in God or deity
An important dimension of spirituality for some individuals is the belief in a God or supreme power or being. This may be a belief in a God who is creator of the world (Judeo–Christian tradition). However, for some individuals their supreme being or deity may be their work or recreational activity. A flexible approach is required since God or deity is defined by the individual.

Ability to express one's own personal beliefs and values
In life there is a fundamental need to express one's own personal beliefs and values. This need is fostered in many modern societies. The inability to express one's own personal beliefs and values can lead to frustration and eventually hostility.

Assessing spiritual needs

Nursing models are now stressing the importance of spiritual needs ('The spiritual variable' described in *The Neuman's systems model* (Neuman 1989) and other nursing models will be discussed in Chapter 3). Case study 2.2 provides an example of a situation where a patient has spiritual needs.

Case study 2.2 Time to think

Jim, 65 years old, was admitted to the ward with a grossly swollen right leg, thigh and calf. A diagnosis of DVT (deep vein thrombosis) was made. He was started on a heparin infusion and kept on total bed rest because of the severe pain when he mobilized.

One morning while the nurse was talking to Jim he became very emotional and began to cry. As the nurse listened to him it emerged

> that on 24 December it was the first anniversary of his wife's death. Jim
> recalled how he had been married for 45 years and for the last 10
> years of his married life had been the main carer for his wife, who
> suffered from rheumatoid arthritis. Jim went on to describe how lonely
> and depressed he felt, stating that a day did not pass without him
> thinking about his wife and the wonderful life they had shared together.
> Jim is not a religious man but he does believe in life after death.
>   Could you identify Jim's spiritual needs?

After reading this case study you probably identified several spiritual needs that Jim was experiencing:

1. Loss of meaning, purpose and fulfilment.
2. The death of his wife and the loss of a very long loving relationship.
3. Jim has lost hope and motivation in his own abilities and the future.
4. There is a need for trust so that Jim can discuss his anxieties and needs in a secure and confidential environment.

Reading this case study illustrates how spiritual needs may present themselves and how they are often interrelated. Jim appears to have lost the ability to find meaning, purpose and fulfilment in his life. The anniversary of his wife's death is approaching and memories and emotions are evoked that remind him that a fundamental part of his life – the relationship and love experienced with his wife – has 'ended'. Jim finds himself alone, isolated and depressed. We may well argue that what Jim is experiencing is a natural grieving process, and correctly so, but Jim is also questioning his life at a very deep level, trying to establish some order and sense so that he can move forward to regain stability. (These issues will be discussed in Chapter 4.)

When addressing spiritual needs there is a need for sensitivity, self-awareness and personal value clarification (we must know ourselves) (Harrison & Burnard 1993) Some individuals' spiritual needs may arise and be developed within a religious framework, as they have a substantive belief in a God or deity and follow the teachings and ideologies of that particular religion. Yet others may find meaning and purpose and value in life by investing energy into relationships, work, hobbies, etc. There are no restrictions or constraints dictating what constitutes a spiritual need. A spiritual need is unique, specifically determined and interpreted or perceived by the individual who demonstrates or expresses that need.

SPIRITUAL DISTRESS

If we all have a spirituality and spiritual needs, then it must follow that when a crisis or sudden event occurs in life we may experience not only physical, psychological and social distress but also spiritual distress. Burnard (1987, p. 377) states that:

Spiritual distress is the result of total inability to invest life with meaning. It can be demotivating, painful and can cause anguish to the sufferer.

This definition or approach implies loss of function, dispiritedness and a recognition of behaviour or feelings that convey an altered spiritual integrity. Labun (1988) has identified seven human experiences that demonstrate an altered spiritual integrity, or spiritual distress: spiritual pain, alienation, anxiety, guilt, anger, loss and despair. These demotivating and debilitating experiences and behaviour suggest that the person becomes dysfunctional, withdrawn, and unable to invest or relate to life in a meaningful and integrating manner. There is a disturbance in the flow of energy from the spiritual dimension to the other dimensions. This loss of equilibrium or disturbance may be the result of several aetiological or contributing factors, some pathophysiological and some situational in origin, for example disease, illness, marital or relationship breakdown, loss/bereavement (think back to Case study 2.2).

If one approaches spiritual development across the lifespan then there are stages within our human development that are often troublesome and confusing, for example adolescence or old age, when one is forced to ask questions and establish meaning (Carson 1989). These periods of questioning and uncertainty in life can result in spiritual distress. If an individual is unable to find meaning in life or the experience causes spiritual pain, spiritual distress, dispiritedness and spiritual collapse, the result may be that the individual experiences inner turmoil, conflict and confusion. There is a need to confer order and find meaning in the situation that has caused the disharmony and distress. From a religious and mystical perspective this period of search and confusion has been called the 'dark night of the soul' described vividly by the Carmelite mystic St John of the Cross.

This classification or category of human experiences has been tentatively recognized as a nursing diagnosis by The National

Group for Classification of Nursing Diagnosis. Carpenito (1982 p. 451) in the book *Nursing Diagnosis: Application to Clinical Practice* describes spiritual distress as:

The state in which the individual experiences or is at risk of experiencing a disturbance in his belief or value system that is his source of strength and hope.

Signs of spiritual distress

The defining characteristics focus primarily upon a disturbance in the individual's belief and value system, which may manifest itself in uncertainty, ambivalence and a sense of emptiness or aloneness. The individual may display other traits such as:

anger
fear
a morbid preoccupation with suffering and death.

As individuals we all search and have a desire to establish order in our life by discovering meaning and purpose. The challenge to the nursing profession is to assist individuals who are spiritually distressed, dispirited, and at times emotionally and physically dysfunctional, to explore life's crisis in an attempt to rediscover meaning and value so that once again they can invest positively in life.

SPIRITUAL WELL-BEING

A logical argument exists in that if we can experience spiritual distress then we must at times experience a sense of spiritual well-being. Hungelmann et al (1985 p. 152) describe spiritual well-being as a state of acceptance of self/others and a positive disposition towards life when they write:

a sense of harmonious interconnectedness between self, others/nature, and ultimate other which exists throughout and beyond time and space. It is achieved through a dynamic and integrative growth process which leads to realisation of the ultimate purpose and meaning of life.

This description implies that in order to experience spiritual well-being an individual must achieve harmonious interconnectedness, peace and acceptance within all dimensions of his or her existence and being as he or she progresses through the different developmental stages and experiences of life. It requires an individual to be introspective and reflective, thus revealing the meaning and the purpose so that consolidation and ultimate acceptance can occur.

Hungelmann et al demonstrate that there is a definite change of focus from the religious (theistic) approaches to spiritual well-being as presented by Byrne, who refers to the definition given by the White House Conference on Aging (cited in Byrne 1985):

the affirmation of life in a relationship with God, self, community and environment which nurtures and celebrates wholeness.

to a realization of a further dimension that has socio-psychological components (Harrison 1993). The above definition implies that there are two distinct, interactive dimensions to spiritual well-being. There is a transcendental or existential relationship with an ultimate other and a purely physio-psychosocial relationship involving the individual with their environment/world and other individuals. These dimensions have been identified by the sociologist Morberg (1971, 1979) and nurse theorist Stoll (1989). They suggest that there is a vertical dimension, referring to the individual's sense of well-being in relation to

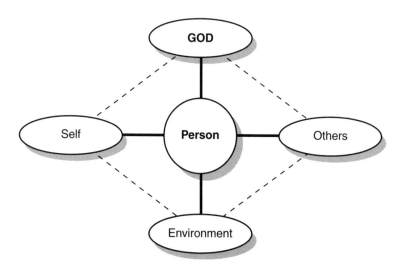

Figure 2.3 The relationship between the horizontal and vertical dimensions of spirituality. (Adapted from Stoll 1989. Reproduced with the permission of W B Saunders.)

their God, and a horizontal dimension, referring to the person's sense of life purpose or satisfaction with their state in the world (Fig. 2.3). This two-dimensional, dualist approach is very similar to the 'conceptual model of the nature of man' developed by Stallwood & Stoll (1975) (discussed in Chapter 3). These approaches to spiritual well-being demonstrate that conceptualization and definition will be difficult because of the numerous factors and variables involved. Nevertheless, this approach emphasizes the interactive and integrative nature of both the vertical and horizontal dimensions, which cannot be viewed in isolation.

Emerging debates

In an attempt to sharpen our understanding, Ellison (1983) proposes that spiritual well-being may not be the same thing as spiritual health. The debate emerging is – are they not the one and same thing? Ellison (1983 p. 332) states:

If we are spiritually healthy we will feel generally alive purposeful, and fulfilled, but only to the extent that we are psychologically healthy as well.

This statement stresses the intimate relationship that spiritual well-being has with the psychological dimension. Yet there exists a danger of misinterpretation since this statement infers that spiritual well-being is determined by our psychological state. It fails to accept spiritual well-being or spirituality as a separate entity, which unifies and integrates in a mystical manner all dimensions of our being. Byrne (1985 p. 32) subscribes to this philosophy when she states:

Emotional support alone will not suffice if the person's problem is spiritual in nature.

Byrne seems to distinguish the spiritual from the emotional and the psychological realms. Reed (1987 p. 336) writes:

spiritual transcendence does not imply a detachment from other dimensions of one's life.

thus emphasizing the unifying and permeating nature of - spirituality. Neuman (1989 p. 29) shares this approach when describing the spiritual variable incorporated in her nursing model:

The author views it as being on a continuum of development that permeates all other client system variables.

Leggieri (1986 p. 50) refers to the integrating approach to spiritual well-being, stating:

Therefore healing must take place on all levels of life because the separate forces work together as an integrated whole within persons.

Spiritual well-being (spiritual health) will be determined by both vertical and horizontal dimensions functioning harmoniously and dynamically together, fostering a positive and meaningful attitude and disposition towards life. Figure 2.3 underlines this dynamic relationship between the person and their relationship with the horizontal and vertical dimensions. In order to have spiritual well-being a person would feel integrated, finding meaning and purpose within both the vertical and the horizontal dimensions. These two dimensions do not function in isolation since to adopt such an approach would be reductionist, suggesting that spirituality is detached from the physical world. These arguments will be further explored in Chapter 3.

By adopting this approach there exists a danger of reducing spiritual well-being to a purely functional, observable and measurable level. If spirituality is transcendent and existential (we have a say in our own destiny), then how can it be reduced to a functional state? Stoll (1989 p. 19) states:

spiritual well-being is not a state but rather is indicative of the presence of spiritual health in the person. Therefore spiritual well-being is identified as behavioural expressions of spiritual health.

Therefore spiritual well-being is not just a functional state but the expression of an underlying state that is the essence and core of one's being. Ellison (1983 p. 332) writes:

If this is an accurate conception we are freed from the burden of trying to exactly or empirically measure the inner contours of one's spirit – a task which is most likely impossible.

All these approaches to the concept of spiritual well-being highlight that there is a need for further clarification, categorization and refinement of the term since conceptual writings on the subject are sparse (Morrison 1989). This will ensure clarity and universality in definition instead of confusion and possible distortion.

Activity 2.4

Having briefly explored the concept of spiritual need, spend a little time reflecting upon your own life and identify any spiritual needs that are important to you.

CONCLUSION

This chapter has explored possible definitions associated with the word spirituality. It has asked you to reflect upon your own understanding of the word in order to clarify meaning and understanding in respect of daily living. Terms associated with spirituality have been discussed and where possible related to nursing practice. The complex and subjective nature of spirituality was revealed and it is suggested that creating an authoritative definition may be difficult. The definitions and arguments developed indicate that spirituality can be applied to all things secular, temporal and mystical. However, there are still many questions that need to be answered if spirituality is to be fully understood and defined.

REFERENCES

Allen C 1991 The inner light. Nursing Standard 5 (20): 52–53
Bradshaw A 1994 Lighting the lamp: the spiritual dimension of nursing care. Scutari Press, London
Bradshaw A 1996 The legacy of Nightingale. Nursing Times 92 (6): 42–43
Burnard P 1987 Spiritual distress and the nursing response: theoretical considerations and counselling skills. Journal of Advanced Nursing 12: 377–382
Burnard P 1988 The spiritual needs of atheists and agnostics. Professional Nurse 4 (3): 130–132
Byrne M 1985 A zest for life! Journal of Gerontological Nursing 11 (4): 30–33
Carpenito L J 1983 Nursing diagnosis: application to clinical practice. J B Lippincott, New York
Carson V B 1989 Spiritual dimensions of nursing practice. W B Saunders, Philadelphia
Colliton M A 1981 The spiritual dimension of nursing. In: Beland I L, Passos J Y (eds) Clinical Nursing, 4th edn. Macmillan, New York
Dickinson C 1975 The search for spiritual meaning. American Journal of Nursing 75 (10): 1789–1793

Dunn P M 1993 An investigation into the concept of spiritual needs of hospitalised patients, from a nursing perspective. Unpublished dissertation, Institute of Nursing Studies, University of Hull, Hull

Ellison W 1983 Spiritual wellbeing: conceptualisation and measurement. Journal of Psychology and Theology 11 (4): 330–340

Erikson H H 1963 Childhood and society, 2nd edn. W W Norton, New York

Frankl V E 1987 Man's search for meaning. An introduction to logotherapy. Hodder & Stoughton, London

Harrison J 1993 Spirituality and nursing practice. Journal of Clinical Nursing 2: 211–217

Harrison J, Burnard P 1993 Spirituality and nursing practice. Avebury, Aldershot

Highfield M F, Cason C 1983 Spiritual needs of patients: are they recognised? Cancer Nursing (June): 187–192

Hungelmann J, Rossi-Kenkel E, Klassen L, Stollenwerk R M 1985 Spiritual well being in older adults: harmonious interconnectedness. Journal of Religion and Health 24 (2): 147–153

Labun E 1988 Spiritual care: an element in nursing care planning. Journal of Advanced Nursing 13: 314–320

Leggieri J 1986 Pastoral care in the hospital: uniqueness and contribution. Topics in Clinical Nursing 8 (2): 47–55

McSherry W 1996 Raising the spirits. Nursing Times 92 (3): 48–49

McSherry W 1997 A descriptive survey of nurses' perceptions of spirituality and spiritual care. Unpublished MPhil thesis, University of Hull, Hull

McSherry W 1998 Nurses' perceptions of spirituality and spiritual care. Nursing Standard 13 (4): 36–40

McSherry W, Draper P 1998 The debates emerging from the literature surrounding the concept of spirituality as applied to nursing. Journal of Advanced Nursing 27: 683–691

Morberg D O 1971 Spiritual well-being: background and issues. White House Conference on Aging, Washington, DC

Morberg D O 1979 Spiritual well-being: sociological perspectives. University Press of America, Washington, DC

Morrison R 1989 Spiritual health care and the nurse. Nursing Standard 4 (13/14): 28–29

Murray R B, Zentner J B 1989 Nursing concepts for health promotion. Prentice Hall, London

Narayanasamy A 1991 Spiritual care: a resource guide. Quay Books, Lancaster

Neuman B 1989 The Neuman systems model, 2nd edn. Appleton & Lange, Norwalk

Reed P G 1987 Spirituality and well-being in terminally-ill hospitalised adults. Research in Nursing and Health 10: 335–344

Reed P G 1992 An emerging paradigm for the investigation of spirituality in nursing. Research in Nursing and Health 15: 349–357

Shelly J A, Fish S 1988 Spiritual care the nurse's role, 3rd edn. Inter Varsity Press, Illinois

Simsen B 1985 Spiritual needs and resources in illness and hospitalisation. Unpublished MSc thesis, University of Manchester, Manchester

Stallwood J, Stoll R 1975 Spiritual dimensions of nursing practice. In: Beland I L, Passos J Y (eds) Clinical Nursing, 3rd edn. Macmillan, New York

Stoll R I 1989 The essence of spirituality. In: Carson V B (ed) Spiritual dimensions of nursing practice. W B Saunders, Philadelphia

Travelbee J 1966 Interpersonal aspects of nursing. Davis, Philadelphia

Turner P 1996 Caring more, doing less. Nursing Times 92 (34): 59–60
Walsh M, Ford P 1988 Nursing rituals: research and rational actions.
    Heinemann Nursing, Oxford
Waugh L A 1992 Spiritual aspects of nursing: a descriptive study of nurses'
    perceptions. Unpublished PhD thesis, Queen Margaret College, Edinburgh
Wright S 1997 Free the spirit. Nursing Times 93 (17): 28–29

FURTHER READING

Exploring the meaning of the word spirituality
These two articles look specifically at the meaning of the word spirituality
and will help develop your knowledge and understanding of the concept.

Cawley N 1997 An exploration of the concept of spirituality. International
    Journal of Palliative Care 3 (1): 31–36
Emblen J D 1992 Religion and spirituality defined according to current use in
    nursing literature. Journal of Professional Nursing 8 (1): 41–47

Explaining the relationship between different religions and spirituality
These authors discuss in some detail the influences that different religions have
had on society and nursing in general.

Burnard P 1988 The spiritual needs of atheists and agnostics. Professional
    Nurse December: 130–132
Gerardi R 1989 Western spirituality and health care. In: Carson V B (ed)
    Spiritual dimensions of nursing practice. W B Saunders, Philadelphia, ch 4,
    p 76
Martin P J 1989 Eastern spirituality and health care. In: Carson V B (ed)
    Spiritual dimensions of nursing practice. W B Saunders, Philadelphia,
    ch 5, p 113
Sampson C 1982 The neglected ethic religious and cultural factors in the care of
    patients. McGraw-Hill, London

General reading
This selection of articles will help to consolidate your understanding of the
term spirituality and its relevance to clinical practice.

Harrison J 1993 Spirituality and nursing practice. Journal of Clinical Nursing 2:
    211–217
McSherry W 1996 Raising the spirits. Nursing Times 92 (3): 48–49
Ross L A 1994 Spiritual aspects of nursing. Journal of Advanced Nursing 19:
    439–447

3

Spirituality within the context of holism

INTRODUCTION

This chapter explores the place that spirituality has within the context of holism. The adjective holistic is used frequently within the caring professions without taking into account its implications. However, consideration needs to be given to what we mean by holism and how the concept may need to be revised to accommodate changing theory and practice. These debates are presented and examined against the emerging literature surrounding spirituality and the provision of spiritual care. The place that spirituality has within the context of nursing theories and models is briefly discussed.

The terms holism and holistic are used frequently by nurses and other health care professionals. Your reflections

Activity 3.1

Spend several minutes reflecting upon the terms holism and holistic. Write down any thought or ideas that come to mind. Think about how you were introduced to these terms and how frequently you hear these words being used.

Box 3.1   The four aspects of holism

Biological
   This refers to the physical and biological process or function of an
   individual essential to maintain life.
Psychological
   Usually implies the cognitive, intellectual, emotional aspects of the
   individual that may shape personality and mental functioning.
Social
   The cultural norms, values and beliefs that influence and classify
   individuals into different groups or communities.
Spiritual
   A vague term used normally to indicate individual's inner beliefs
   commonly related to religious affiliation or belief in the existence of
   a God or supreme power.

---

may have revealed that these terms are associated with
treating the 'whole' person or providing care that seeks
to address all the dimensions of an individual's life, for
example the physical, social, psychological and spiritual
(Box 3.1).

You were probably introduced to these terms during your
nurse education. Alternatively you may have heard the words
being used in practice or read them incorporated within a ward
philosophy of care or nursing textbook.

If you had been asked to draw a diagram that represents
holism then you may well have drawn one similar to Figure 3.1.
The circle represents the 'whole' person while the four different
quarters, described earlier (Box 3.1), represent fundamental
dimensions. However, this could be classified as a reductionist
approach because there is no indication that all four quarters or
dimensions are interrelated or dependent upon each other. The
diagram reduces the whole into manageable mechanistic
units. The diagrammatic representation is void of any interaction or interconnection between the individual, his or her environment or with other people – indeed the whole of creation. It
assumes that individuals function in isolation. Each aspect of
our being is placed into a functional box not overlapping the
next (as shown by the black solid lines). Holism is represented
in a very narrow insular way. This raises two important
questions:

What is holism?
How has the concept been defined within nursing?

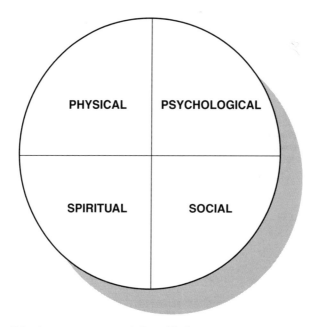

Figure 3.1   A common representation of holism.

HOLISM

The word 'holism' originates from the Greek word *holos*, meaning whole (Griffin 1993, Ham-Ying 1993). The term holism implies that all dimensions of our lives are all equally important to our functioning and well-being: 'The whole is greater than the sum of its parts' (Patterson 1998). Yet your reflection reveals that the biological and medical models of care contradict the term since they separate individuals into functional mechanistic units or biological systems (discussed in Chapter 1), often at the expense of seeing the whole person and his or her situation (see Box 3.2).

Several authors (Buckle 1993, Griffin 1993, Kolcaba 1997, Patterson 1998) have explored and discussed the term holism and their conclusions indicate there may be no single definition because the term is vague and difficult to pin down.

Ham-Ying (1993) implies that nurses do not have an adequate understanding of the concept of holism, nor a sufficient educational preparation, and the result may be that holistic care will

---

Box 3.2 Definitions of holism, holistic and reductionism

Holism
  The individual is perceived as a 'whole'. There is acknowledgement that all systems – biological, psychosocial, spiritual and environmental – cannot be viewed in isolation because they all 'make up the whole person'.
Holistic
  Attending to all dimensions of an individual with equal importance.
Reductionism
  The tendency to reduce or divide individuals into functional mechanist units. This is the opposite of holism.

---

not be fully operational within the context of nursing practice. With this point in mind it might be useful to discuss how the term is defined within nursing.

The Churchill Livingstone (1996 p. 176) *Dictionary of nursing* does not offer a definition of holism but defines holistic as:

In a nursing context, caring for the whole patient ⇒total patient care.

This definition reinforces the notion that holistic care concerns the entire person. A possible reason why these terms are open to misinterpretation is because, like spirituality, a great deal of uncertainty still surrounds them. Buckle (1993) argues that the term holism is used inaccurately because it is used interchangeably with the word complementary, thus underlining the confusion and misconceptions surrounding the use of the term. From this brief analysis of the term holism, it would appear that there is some degree of ambiguity about the precise meaning of the word. Despite these uncertainties, the relevance and benefits of using these terms in the provision of health and nursing care cannot be dismissed. Holism is a common feature in many nursing models (Pearson & Vaughan 1986) and has guided and shaped the direction of nursing care throughout its inception and evolution.

In summary, the word holism is used to describe the 'whole' and the adjective holistic is used to describe the application of the term to practice, for example the provision of holistic care. There is recognition that all parts of an individual share equal importance in a balanced manner. If we are providing holistic care then we attend to all dimensions of an individual, giving each the same amount of importance.

REDUCTIONISM

A reductionist approach would be to reduce the individual into manageable units. Roper et al's (1980) nursing model could be classified as a reductionist model because it divides the individual into a set of systems or activities that are required for daily living, such as breathing, elimination, eating and drinking, and sexuality. Yet the reality is that all these systems are related to and dependent upon each other. A purely reductionist approach focuses upon specific aspects of the person without giving due consideration to the other dimensions and their relationships with each other. However, clinical experience shows that there may be some benefits from implementing a reductionist approach. Different aspects of care can be delegated and managed by the appropriate professionals. It would appear that this approach to patient management is used in many health care settings. This is illustrated by the following case study.

Case study 3.1

A middle-aged man with Type I diabetes mellitus is admitted with a 'diabetic foot'. He has a large ulcer affecting his right big toe and is unable to cope at home with his illness. The man complains that his life has been altered dramatically by the condition.

 Activity 3.2

Spend several minutes reflecting upon this man's situation and write down how a reductionist approach might address the problems of the diabetic foot and other issues the man is experiencing.

The chances are you identified a number of professionals who may be asked to contribute to this man's care needs (Box 3.3).

Closer inspection of the list reveals how reductionism delegates areas of responsibility to other professionals. It could still

> **Box 3.3** How reductionism addresses the 'whole' – achieving total patient care
>
> | | |
> |---|---|
> | Doctors | Overall management of medical care |
> | Nurses | Overall responsibility for nursing care interventions |
> | Dietician | Nutritional support |
> | Podiatrist | Management of diabetic foot |
> | Occupational therapist | Adaptation and adjustment in activities of living |
> | Religious/spiritual leader | Religious and spiritual needs |
> | Social worker | Advice on support services available |
> | Physiotherapist | Mobility |
> | Diabetes specialist nurse | Advice concerning management of diabetes |

be said that the man is receiving 'holistic care' or total patient care, because the key aspects are being addressed. Problems with this approach are that a breakdown in communication can mean that important information is not communicated. Likewise professionals may only focus upon their own specific area of responsibility, which can sometimes mean that problems the patient may have remain undetected. The greatest danger is that care can appear fragmented and an holistic perspective of how the different dimensions affect and are affected by each other is lost. Some nursing areas remove this risk by holding multidisciplinary or case conferences where information is exchanged, progress discussed and further interventions decided.

NURSING MODELS: A BRIEF OVERVIEW

It is not the intention of this chapter to provide a detailed analysis of all the nursing models that have been developed; that is beyond the scope of this book. However, there are several texts available that provide a detailed account of such models (Walsh 1991). This section will look at the place that spirituality has within some of these models, demonstrating how the growing awareness of the importance of spirituality to an individual's sense of well-being has led some theorists to revisit and revise their theories to incorporate the spiritual dimension (Neuman 1995).

Activity 3.3

Spend some time reflecting upon any nursing models that you have heard about or used in practice. Write down your understanding of the model, paying particular attention to any aspect of spirituality that it might address.

Undertaking Activity 3.3 may have proved difficult for two main reasons. First, our knowledge of nursing models is dependent upon two fundamental factors:

The models we have been introduced to during our nurse education. Related to this is the manner in which they were taught and applied to practice. Often if they are taught very theoretically and not applied you can be left more confused, finding it difficult to see the relevance of such material.

The regularity with which we use or encounter such models within practice.

Second, within the UK we are normally introduced to a small range of theories and models. It could be argued that the teaching of nursing theories and models is purely an academic exercise. The relevance of such knowledge received may not be directly relevant to one's area of practice (unless the area in which we work uses the particular model(s) being presented as a framework for care delivery). Therefore within the UK you may only have educational and practical experience in the use of the 'model of daily living' because this has been developed by British nurse theorists and is widely acknowledged and used in clinical practice.

What is a nursing model?

A nursing model represents a personal view of how individuals are made, function and interact with the world. Walsh (1991 p. 8) summarizes:

Nursing models, therefore, are not watertight theories, but rather sets of ideas about the way patients and nurses interact. The dangers of reductionism and losing touch with reality are such that model development must take place with at least one foot in the real world of practical nursing care.

Therefore models represent the world of nursing from different perspectives, offering a set of ideas or a framework for the delivery of care. Conceptual models of nursing present a set of ideas concerning the way that individuals may live, react to illness or interact with their world. It must be stressed that they represent only one world view. For example Orem's (1985) theories concerning self-care or Neuman's (1995) systems model address the different systems involved in people's reaction to health and illness. It could even be argued that there are as many nursing models as there are thinking nurses, since we all have our own individual and personal philosophies concerning what makes us think, feel and react differently to stressful situations.

These points bring into question the direct relevance and purpose of nursing models in the delivery of nursing. Walsh (1991) believes nursing models are useful because they provide structure and direction in the provision of care, while other authors are very sceptical and critical of their relevance to nursing (Luker 1988, Cash 1990, Draper 1990, Kenny 1993). Despite recent criticism of nursing models (Tierney 1998), it would appear that they are here to stay.

SPIRITUALITY AND NURSING MODELS

It was stated earlier that the majority of nursing models embrace an holistic approach. If this statement were accurate, then most nursing models by their very nature should address the concept of spirituality explicitly within their theories and frameworks. Recent debates indicate that this is not the case and only a minority of nursing models incorporate or address the spiritual nature of individuals. Oldnall (1995 p. 418) provides some reasons why the spiritual dimension is not adequately addressed within nursing theories:

Perhaps one reason why nursing models and theories do not appear to work in clinical practice is because they have evolved in the echelons of academia and have been devolved down to the practitioners to operationalize at a clinical level. This may explain, to some degree, why the concept of spirituality has been omitted totally, or at least not developed sufficiently, in existing theories and models.

Oldnall implies that the assumption that most nursing models have an holistic approach to care is inaccurate and misguided. If nursing models and theories embraced holism, then they would address the spiritual dimension. Oldnall (1995, 1996) implies that there needs to be cultural shift – a change in emphasis. Models should not be solely developed in the 'ivory towers of academia' and then be expected to work in practice. This top-down approach to theory development may overlook and fail to incorporate many issues that are being faced by nurses working on the front line. This approach may have prevented the spiritual dimension from being incorporated within contemporary nursing theories and models.

It appears that the academic era of nursing is being challenged within the UK and the change in emphasis that has been sought by chief nurses and those in practice has arrived. In the mid-1980s there was a move to improve the educational and professional credibility of nursing by integrating it within universities. However, recent discontent and levels of dissatisfaction by managers in practice has resulted in a change of opinion. In the Government's new document *Making a difference: strengthening the nursing, midwifery and health visiting contribution to health and health care* (Department of Health 1999) the need for education and practice to work more closely in the education and training of student nurses is underlined. The pendulum has swung to the other end and it would seem that National Health Service trusts now have a greater say in the education of student nurses. This approach is of particular importance to matters concerning spirituality and the provision of spiritual care.

Importantly, this shift in emphasis must be reflected in subsequent theory development. There is a need to have a 'bottom-up' approach whereby practice is put into theory, or theories and models will remain detached from practice and in the realm of academics or theorists.

Caution

If the concerns of those in practice relating to this dimension of care are not listened to, then any attempt to develop this aspect of care will remain an academic exercise unrelated to and divorced from the reality of practice.

What do the theorists have to say?

Martsolf & Mickley (1998) present a review of modern nurse theorists' ideas concerning spirituality. After reviewing the contribution to nursing knowledge made by some of the contemporary nurse theorists, Martsolf & Mickley indicate the position that spirituality has within those ideas. This section offers a summary of the information provided in Martsolf & Mickley (1998). It is beyond the scope of this book to provide a full critique of the place spirituality holds within each model. Therefore this section will only indicate whether the model addresses the spiritual dimension explicitly or implicitly (as defined in Box 3.4) and provide a very brief outline of how spirituality is addressed by a particular theorist (Boxes 3.5 and 3.6).

Many nurse theorists acknowledge the place that spirituality has within the context of holism. Whether the spiritual dimension is explicit or implicit within the theory, this indicates a growing realization of the importance of the dimension to a sense of well-being and completeness. The models reinforce the need for the spiritual dimension to be considered in both an individual and a global sense. The spirituality of an individual is influenced and shaped by many factors: environmental, internal, political and social. To view spirituality purely as a theory in its own right would be divisive and reductionist. There is a need to be aware of the many systems and forces, both positive and negative, that can shape an individual's sense of health and total well-being. The theories and models indicate that individuals are made up of many systems interacting with each other. These systems work in harmony to maintain equilibrium. Many forces or stressors can affect the individual's state. These forces can be internal or

---

Box 3.4 The terms defined

Explicitly
 There is clear mention or reference to the importance of the concept.
  Removal of the spiritual element would have an impact upon the theory.
Implicitly
 Reference to the spiritual dimension is inferred in the theories and concepts of the model or addressed as a subcomponent.
  However, removal of the spiritual element would have no influence on the theory.

external. It is the individual's ability to adapt or restore balance when affected by such forces that results in illness or restoration to wholeness. The nurse's role is to assist in this process of restoration. If restoration cannot be achieved, then it is the nurse's role to prepare the individual for a dignified death.

The theorists' work highlights the complex nature of human organisms and how we are interdependent and interconnected with others, the wider community, and ourselves. Nursing theories and models alert us to the fact that spirituality is an integral aspect of the individual's lived, total experience. It operates and pervades all levels of an individual's existence from the cradle to the grave. The theories reveal that the

---

Box 3.5   Spirituality implicit within the theory or model

Rogers (1980)
This model considers 'unitary human beings'. The word spirituality was not used directly in the work addressing the science of unitary human beings, but has been attached to aspects of the theory by other authors (Smith 1994).

Levine (1967)
This model has 'four conservation principles' and considers that we are adaptive beings in a state of interaction with our environment, both inner and external. The external environment consists of three key components: perceptual, operational and conceptual. It is within the conceptual that reference is made to spirituality.

Roy (1980)
Called the 'adaptation model', this model considers the moral, ethical and spiritual self. This aspect of Roy's model helps the individual to answer questions in relation to belief and existence.

Leininger (1991)
The concepts of 'cultural care theory' are central to Leininger's work. It could be argued that spirituality is loosely addressed in connection with the religious influences upon which different cultures are formed.

Johnson (1980)
The 'behavioural systems' model indicates that we have a specific set of response patterns that act together to form an integrated whole. The behavioural system comprises several subsystems. It is within these subsystems that spirituality may feature. One subsystem is affiliation – the need to relate to one's own beliefs such as the belief in a God.

Roper et al (1990)
Early editions of *The elements of nursing* did not give recognition to the spiritual dimension. However, by the third edition there is realization of the place that spirituality may have with regard to the well-being of individuals. Spirituality is not addressed explicitly but rather within the context of religion and culture (Bradshaw 1994).

Box 3.6   Spirituality explicit within the theory/model

Neuman (1995)
   The 'Neuman's systems model' includes the spiritual variable. Neuman
   indicates that the patient may not have a conscious awareness of
   this component but it is present in all individuals. The spiritual
   variable has the potential to influence the individuals systems
   positively. Spiritual awareness may be developed at any time
   during the lifespan.

Newman (1986)
   Newman's 'model of health' assumes that health is associated with
   the expansion of an individual's consciousness. Spirituality is used
   broadly in connection with human interactions.

Parse (1981)
   In the *Man–living–health* theory the term spirituality is not used.
   However, one of the theoretical principles of this theory is that
   individuals can choose personal meaning. Therefore if the concept
   were removed from Parse's theory the work would be adversely
   affected.

Watson (1985)
   This philosophy and science of human caring operates around nurse
   and patient interactions. The spiritual dimension of the individual is
   acknowledged. The goal of nursing is to enable individuals to
   achieve a balance between mind, body and spirit, finding meaning
   in their existence.

---

spiritual dimension is important at behavioural levels – our
interactions with the environment and others. It is concerned
with each person's ability to find meaning and purpose in situations and events. It enables us to achieve or reach our opti-
mum potential.

Those nursing theories and models that omit the spiritual
dimension are failing to address a fundamental concept. The
omission fails to recognize the impact that a loss of spiritual
well-being might have on the overall quality of life and sense of
well-being experienced by an individual. The absence of the
spiritual dimension may not be a conscious omission but rather
a preoccupation with the political, economic, educational and
social influences that prevailed at the time of construction. The
absence of spirituality within some models may reflect the theorists' inability to appreciate or critically appraise material used
in their theory development. Bradshaw (1994 p. 188) shares this
view:

But this analysis has also highlighted a further problem in nursing
theory. That is, not only do nursing theories uncritically incorporate

concepts from other academic disciplines without reference to their philosophical background, context, and coherence, but they also employ insights and arguments from fellow nurses without critically examining or even addressing the source of their positions.

Interestingly, this argument is directed towards an attempt by Roper et al (1990) to address the concept of spirituality within their model of nursing. The point reinforces the need for theorists to appraise critically existing knowledge before incorporating it within subsequent revision.

This brief review of theories and models indicates that the spiritual dimension has an important place within the context of holism. The spiritual dimension as represented in several of the nursing theories seems to be a force that brings unity and harmony to the human state.

Food for thought

Before academics, and indeed practitioners, accuse theorists who fail to acknowledge the spiritual dimension of being misguided and lacking spiritual awareness, we must consider the full picture. It may be the era and social context in which theories are constructed and tested that determines individuals' thinking and assumptions. It will be interesting to review nursing theories that are currently being constructed in a time of spiritual reawakening.

SPIRITUALITY AS A UNIFYING FORCE

In Chapter 2 the analogy of spirituality as a football was made, stressing that it is a force that pervades, integrates and interconnects all aspects of our existence and being. It has been suggested in the previous section that spirituality is a force that brings unity and stability to our being. Surveying nurse perceptions of spirituality, McSherry (1997 p. 120) writes:

Of the nurses surveyed (276) 50.3% felt that spirituality was a unifying force which enabled individuals to be at peace with oneself and the world. This finding suggests that nurses see spirituality originating from within themselves A force which brings unity and harmony. This finding implies that nurses are aware that spirituality is multi-dimensional which is related to the natural and supernatural dimensions of existence. These would be the Vertical and Horizontal dimensions as defined by Stoll (1989).

The research findings suggest that nurses perceive spirituality as something that influences the physical, psychological and social aspects of our being in an integrated manner. Spirituality is an invisible force that brings unity and harmony to self, others and the larger universe. The spiritual dimension is a mysterious and transcendent force that assists the individual in finding meaning, purpose and fulfilment. It is a force that transcends the rational and intellectual capabilities of our human state, uniting us with the whole of creation both at a material and supernatural level.

MODELS REPRESENTING THE SPIRITUAL DIMENSION

Stoll (1989) uses a two-dimensional approach to show the relationship between the spiritual dimension and other aspects of our lives (Fig. 3.2). She uses a vertical line to show the individual's connection with the mystical–transcendental domain. This relationship may consist of a belief in a supreme being or God. The supreme being may be values or principles that guide the person's life. A horizontal line is used to describe the relationship that exists between self and others. An inner circle is used to depict the person and his or her relationship with both vertical and horizontal dimensions. Stoll stresses the interrelatedness and interconnectedness of all the dimensions by the use of dashed lines. Three spiritual needs operating within the model are the needs for love, forgiveness and trust. For Stoll spirituality is developed throughout life and the dimension may come into focus during times of health and illness.

One major limitation of this approach is that it separates the different dimensions. For example, the vertical line representing the mystical is not integrated with the psychosocial or environmental. The model does not seem to stress the unifying nature and intimacy that spirituality has with all the different aspects of a person's life. The model could be described as dualistic and functionalist because it implies that spirituality serves a specific need, for example the need for love, trust and forgiveness (Shelly & Fish 1988, McSherry & Draper 1998). If these needs are met, then the person will have meaning, purpose and fulfilment in life.

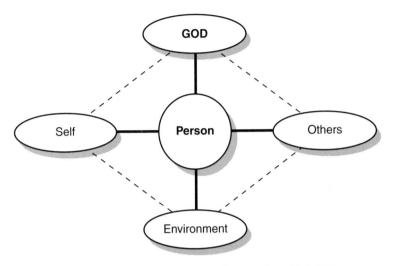

Figure 3.2   Stoll's two-dimensional model. (Adapted from Stoll 1989. Reproduced with permission of W B Saunders.)

In Chapter 2 the 'conceptual model of the nature of man' described by Stallwood & Stoll (1975) was mentioned. This model, illustrated in Figure 3.3, emphasizes the integrated nature of individuals and illustrates clearly the place that spirituality has within the context of holism. Unlike Stoll's two-dimensional

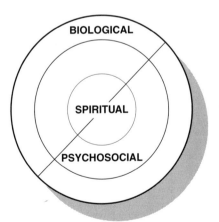

Figure 3.3   Stallwood & Stoll's (1975) conceptual model of the nature of humans. (Reprinted with the permission of Scribner, a Division of Simon & Schuster from CLINICAL NURSING 3/e by Irene L Beland and J Y Passos. Copyright © 1975 Macmillan Publishing Company.)

approach, this model represents simply the relationship between the physical, psychosocial and spiritual, indicating that spirituality expresses itself via the total being.

In this model the outermost circle represents the physical body – the biological world. This is the body as seen by others and self. The physical body enables individuals to relate to the world via the five main senses of touch, taste, hearing, sight and smell. The second circle depicts the psychosocial dimension. This is the part of the person associated with self-consciousness, personality, intellect, moral senses and will. It could be argued that the psychological aspects are influenced and shaped by the social context and environmental and cultural influences. The innermost circle is described as spiritual. It is hard to define and comprehend and is therefore mysterious. The spirit pervades all other dimensions of the individual. Within the spiritual realm is the potential for awareness of God – however that is defined by the individual. The inner circle

---

Case study 3.2 A sense of guilt

James is 47 years of age. He was admitted onto an acute psychiatric admissions unit for depression resulting in weight loss for which no pathology had been diagnosed. On admission he looked very anxious and withdrawn. He communicated with staff as a matter of courtesy but did not really identify or relate to any other patients on the unit. The admitting nurse found it difficult to assess James' mental status. He used one-word answers and did not really disclose much about himself or the recent problems that he has been experiencing. His entire body language used closed postures – indicating further his reluctance for anyone to come close. James has been married for 20 years and his wife cannot comprehend the change in personality that he is displaying. Several months earlier they had a loving and open relationship. Several days passed and James appeared more relaxed and less threatened by his admission into the unit. He started to communicate more easily with all staff and other patients on the unit.

In the course of a conversation with one of the nurses James disclosed the source of his anxiety. He recalls that several years earlier a friend had introduced him to the gambling circuit. In recent months the friend had been threatening to reveal James's hidden secret to his wife. Since this revelation James had been unable to sleep. He had become preoccupied with the repercussions of this upon his marriage and family. Now he felt very guilty and anxious about the entire situation, becoming increasingly depressed. As the months passed and the blackmail intensified he felt more trapped and isolated. Eventually he met the ransom by paying the friend several thousand pounds – severing his ties with gambling and the friend in an attempt to preserve his relationships.

represents the vertical line in Stoll's two-dimensional model. The broken lines in the diagram indicate that individuals function as a 'whole'.

The physical body (outer circle) influences the psychosocial and spiritual dimensions. The psychosocial (second circle) expresses itself through the physical, while the spiritual pervades every aspect of an individual's total being. In essence the human spirit unifies the whole person.

The way in which all these dimensions are interconnected and interdependent can be illustrated by a case study (Case study 3.2).

The case study illustrates how the different circles are all interrelated and interconnected. James had begun to experience physical symptoms as a result of the unrest and loss of stability in the spiritual and psychosocial domains. The sense of guilt he experienced was disrupting the flow of energy and stability in all aspects of his life. The cumulative effect of his addiction was the manifestation of depression accompanied by nausea and vomiting. James' entire being had been affected by the spiritual, psychosocial stressors. This case study illustrates simply Stallwood & Stoll's (1975) conceptual model of the nature of humans.

A limitation of the Stallwood & Stoll model is the over preoccupation with the intellectual and moral cognitive functioning of the individual. The model implies that a functioning intellect is a necessity to the development of spirituality. This issue is explored further in the next section.

Activity 3.4

Spend several minutes reflecting upon the two different models presented in this section. Write down any thoughts, ideas or concerns that you might have about spirituality and holism.

PSYCHOLOGICAL AND SPIRITUAL

When I am presenting workshops or lectures concerning spirituality one question that is continually asked is: How do you distinguish the spiritual from the psychological?

My immediate response is to sigh and take a deep breath before attempting to offer an explanation or an illustration.

However, this question is extremely important and worthy of further explanation. It is true that many of the things associated with spirituality such as our need to find meaning, purpose and fulfilment are directly related to our psychological well-being. The danger is to reduce and separate our spiritual needs and psychological needs into different domains or categories. Spirituality is not a separate entity that can be turned on or off at the touch of a switch because it is continually present, whether we are conscious of this or not. This point is highlighted in Case study 3.3.

Case study 3.3   Psychological and spiritual

Martha is 56 years old. At the age of 50 she was diagnosed with pre-senile dementia. The signs and symptoms had been associated with stress. However a CT scan confirmed organic changes and the diagnosis. Prior to her diagnosis she had been a highly successful businesswoman. Her final position was director of a large international company. Despite being successful Martha had a strong belief and faith in a God but did not attend any formal religious organization.

In her spare time Martha had enjoyed a range of activities such as travel, painting and regular cross-country runs in the country. Martha liked to spend time on her own reflecting and keeping in touch with the creative aspects of her personality. The slow progression of the disease meant that Martha was very much aware of the deteriorative nature of the illness and the result that this might have upon her life. As the disease progressed she was unable to maintain her interests and activities. She became withdrawn and isolated within her own inner world. Familiar faces and locations lost their meaning. Martha's modesty and privacy were lost as she began to become incontinent. Her entire personality changed, resulting in aggressive outbursts, and on several occasions household objects were thrown around the room. Martha had become the complete opposite to everything in which she believed.

Having read this case study you are probably wondering what this has to do with the psychological and spiritual debate. One important question that needs to be asked to help us make sense of this situation is: Has Martha's spirituality changed as a result of the progressive disease?

Martha is still the same person with all her personal beliefs and values. What has changed is her psychological functioning and processes. Fundamentally Martha is still the same individual, but her cognitive processes and physiological functions have been disrupted by this degenerative disorder. It is not the intention of this chapter to enter into deep philosophical debate. However, I would argue that Martha still has the same spirituality and even among the inner turmoil she is a spiritual being who possesses spiritual needs that require spiritual care.

This case study highlights the fact that spirituality pervades all dimensions of one's existence in a meaningful and intricate manner, whether there is a conscious awareness of this or not. Spirituality and the spiritual dimension still exist in the absence of a functioning intellect or other psychological processes. This point contradicts Stallwood & Stoll (1975 p. 1088), who write:

An individual may choose which components will be master (god, controlling force) of his person – the body, the intellect, the emotion, the will, the moral sense, or the spirit.

The same principles implicit in Martha's situation can be applied to individuals with severe learning disabilities or any other condition that affects psychological function or reasoning. Tournier (1954) indicates that the spirit expresses itself through the physical and psychological aspects of our lives but it is neither physical nor psychological. Therefore we can conclude by saying that spirituality is of another dimension that transcends nature. It is something very mysterious but real.

WHAT IS THE RELEVANCE TO NURSING PRACTICE?

This chapter has been very abstract in that it has addressed the concepts of holism and spirituality in theoretical and academic terms. The material has probably left you asking yourself a fundamental question: What are the implications of all this for nursing practice?

The material presented in this chapter reveals that the concepts of holism and spirituality are very complex and subjective. It would appear that there is no single authoritative definition for either word. The brief exploration of spirituality within the context of nursing theories and models suggests that spirituality is a fundamental part of what makes individuals experience health and an overall sense of well-being. Yet some of the points raised in this chapter warrant further clarification

---

Box 3.7 Implications for practice

Ambiguity in definition of holism and spirituality – implications for practice.
Models of nursing and the absence of spirituality within them.
Application of theory into practice and vice versa – practice into theory.
A need to generate theory that addresses the spiritual dimension in that it reflects the concerns of practitioners.

---

because they have important implications for practice. These points are presented above in Box 3.7.

The chapter has demonstrated that there still exists some ambiguity and misconception surrounding the words holism and holistic. When using the term holism all aspects of an individual must be consider, both micro (concerning the individual) and macro (concerning the wider context such as political, economic and environmental factors). When applying the terms to practice consideration must be given to more than just the physical, psychological, social and spiritual. A narrow definition does not recognize the interconnectedness or interdependence of the different domains.

Nursing models demonstrate the uniqueness and complex nature of individuals. However, such theories must incorporate the concerns of those who have to use these models in practice. Theory development must also arise from within practice – instead of being devised and articulated in the realms of academia and thrust upon the practitioner. The need to listen to practitioners is evident in the recently published document *Fitness for practice* (UKCC 1999). Senior nurses and educationalists throughout the UK have identified a deficit in the ability of newly qualified nurses to provide the most fundamental of care. Through voicing their concerns they have managed to bring about possible reform and ultimately change in the way in which nurses will be educated.

The same principle needs to be applied to nursing theories and models. Practitioners who are directly involved in care delivery are indicating a deficit in some of the models because they do not address the spiritual dimension. Subsequent theory development or revision needs to incorporate these concerns and address the omission. There needs to be a bottom-up and a top-down approach to theory development like the formation of stalactites and stalagmites in a dark cave. The process of integrating theory and practice will only be complete when both can work together, just like the stalactite and stalagmite fusing together. However, the process of fusion in the dark cave will take many decades. The luxury of time is not available to the nursing profession because the situation will arise where theory does not reflect practice and vice versa. It is evident that practitioners are aware of the need to attend to individual spiritual needs. This should now be reflected in the content of nursing curricula.

CONCLUSION

This chapter has demonstrated the place that spirituality has within the context of holism. A brief overview of the place that spirituality has within some nursing models has been provided. However, this analysis is very simplistic and not comprehensive. Yet the information indicates that there is an urgent need for theory and practice to unite. Some of these issues concerning the place of spirituality with the context of holism will rumble on for many more years. It is apparent that spirituality does have an important and central place within human existence. The challenge to the nursing profession is to reach a consensus and common vocabulary when addressing the two important issues of holism and spirituality. Until such a time the spiritual dimension will remain an elusive, mysterious aspect of human existence.

Final thought

Do you think a consensus will be reached by nurse theorists and practitioners about the exact role that spirituality plays within people's lives?

REFERENCES

Bradshaw A 1994 Lighting the lamp: the spiritual dimension of nursing care. Scutari Press, London
Buckle J 1993 When is holism not complementary? British Journal of Nursing 2 (15): 744–745

Cash K 1990 Nursing models and the idea of nursing. International Journal of Nursing Studies 27 (3): 249–256

Churchill Livingstone 1996 Churchill Livingstone's dictionary of nursing, 17th edn. Churchill Livingstone, Edinburgh

Department of Health 1999 Making a difference: strengthening the nursing, midwifery and health visiting contribution to health and health care. Department of Health, London

Draper P 1990 The development of theory in British nursing: current position and future prospects. Journal of Advanced Nursing 15: 12–15

Griffin A 1993 Holism in nursing: its meaning and value. British Journal of Nursing 2 (6): 310–312

Ham-Ying S 1993 Analysis of the concept of holism within the context of nursing. British Journal of Nursing 2 (15): 771–775

Johnson D E 1980 The behavioural systems model for nursing. In: Riehl J P, Roy C (eds) Conceptual models for nursing practice, 2nd edn. Appleton-Century-Crofts, New York

Kenny T 1993 Nursing models fail in practice. British Journal of Nursing 2: 133–136

Kolcaba R 1997 The primary holisms in nursing. Journal of Advanced Nursing 25: 290–296

Leininger M M 1991 Cultural care diversity and universality: a theory of nursing. National League for Nursing Press, New York

Levine M E 1967 The four conservation principles of nursing. Nursing Forum 6 (1): 45–49

Luker K 1988 Do models work? Nursing Times 88 (5): 27–28

Martsolf D S, Mickley J R 1998 The concept of spirituality in nursing theories: differing world-views and extent of focus. Journal of Advanced Nursing 27: 294–303

McSherry W 1997 A descriptive survey of nurses' perceptions of spirituality and spiritual care. Unpublished MPhil thesis, University of Hull, Hull

McSherry W, Draper P 1998 The debates emerging from the literature surrounding the concept of spirituality as applied to nursing. Journal of Advanced Nursing 27: 683–691

Neuman B 1995 The Neuman systems model, 3rd edn. Appleton & Lange, Norwalk

Newman M A 1986 Health as expanding consciousness. CV Mosby, St Louis

Oldnall A 1996 A critical analysis of nursing: meeting the spiritual needs of patients. Journal of Advanced Nursing 23: 138–144

Oldnall A S 1995 On the absence of spirituality in nursing theories and models. Journal of Advanced Nursing 21: 417–418

Orem D E 1985 Nursing: concepts of practice, 3rd edn. McGraw-Hill, New York

Parse R R 1981 Man–living–health: a theory of nursing. John Wiley, New York

Patterson E F 1998 The philosophy and physics of holistic health care: spiritual healing as a workable interpretation. Journal of Advanced Nursing 27: 287–293

Pearson A, Vaughan B 1986 Nursing models for practice. Heinemann, London

Rogers M E 1980 Nursing: a science of unitary man. In: Riehl J P, Roy C (eds) Conceptual models for nursing practice, 2nd edn. Appleton-Century-Crofts, New York

Roper N, Logan W, Tierney A (1980) The elements of nursing: a model for nursing based on a model of living, 2nd edn. Churchill Livingstone, Edinburgh

Roper N, Logan W, Tierney A (1990) The elements of nursing: a model for nursing based on a model of living, 3rd edn. Churchill Livingstone, Edinburgh

Roy C 1980 The Roy adaptation model. In: Riehl J P, Roy C (eds) Conceptual models for nursing practice, 2nd edn. Appleton-Century-Crofts, New York

Shelly J A, Fish S 1988 Spiritual care: the nurse's role, 3rd edn. Inter Varsity Press, Illinois

Smith D W 1994 Toward developing a theory of spirituality. Visions 2 (1): 35–43

Stallwood J, Stoll R 1975 Spiritual dimensions of nursing practice. In: Beland I J, Passos J Y (eds) Clinical nursing, 3rd edn. Macmillan, New York

Stoll R I 1989 The essence of spirituality. In: Carson V B (ed) Spiritual dimensions of nursing practice. W B Saunders, Philadelphia

Tierney A J 1998 Nursing models: extant or extinct? Journal of Advanced Nursing 28 (1): 77–85

Tournier P 1954 A doctor's case book in the light of the Bible. SCM Press, London

UKCC (1999) Fitness for practice. The UKCC Commission for Nursing and Midwifery Education. United Kingdom Central Council for Nursing, Midwifery and Health Visiting, London

Walsh M 1991 Models in clinical nursing – the way forward. Baillière Tindall, London

Watson J 1985 Nursing: human science and human care: a theory of nursing. Appleton-Century-Crofts, Norwalk

---

FURTHER READING

The concept of holism
These texts will provide you with an insight into the concept of holism as applied to nursing.

Buckle J 1993 When is holism not complementary? British Journal of Nursing 2 (15): 744–745

Griffin A 1993 Holism in nursing: its meaning and value. British Journal of Nursing 2 (6): 310–312

Ham-Ying S 1993 Analysis of the concept of holism within the context of nursing. British Journal of Nursing 2 (15): 771–775

Absence of models
Oldnall's work will introduce you to the debates surrounding the absence of spirituality within nursing theories and models.

Oldnall A S 1995 On the absence of spirituality in nursing theories and models. Journal of Advanced Nursing 21: 417–418

Models representing spirituality
By reading the work of these two authors you will gain a deeper understanding of the two models presented in this chapter.

Stallwood J, Stoll R 1975 Spiritual dimensions of nursing practice. In: Beland I J, Passos J Y (eds) Clinical nursing, 3rd edn. Macmillan, New York

Stoll R I 1989 The essence of spirituality. In: Carson V (ed) Spiritual dimensions of nursing practice. W B Saunders, Philadelphia

4

Providing spiritual care using the nursing process

INTRODUCTION

Chapter 2 explored the concept of spirituality, offering several explanations and definitions. These definitions were revisited in Chapter 3 when the concept of spirituality was discussed in relation to holism and conceptual models of care. This chapter covers the concept of spirituality in relation to the 'nursing process', identifying how spiritual care can be provided within this framework. It is important to remember that individuals who come into hospital will arrive with their own spirituality and spiritual needs that have developed across their lifespan.

It is wrong to imagine that a person's spirituality, or indeed their spiritual needs, will be left at the entrance of the hospital or outside the care setting. In fact Murray & Zentner's (1989) definition of spirituality suggests that for some patients illness or hospitalization may see a refocusing or questioning of their spirituality. An illness, or indeed any crisis, may act as a trigger that moves the individual to revisit, encounter, or 'get in touch with' their own spirituality (Narayanasamy 1996). Therefore it is not unrealistic to assume that at some point during the course of a nurse's professional practice he or she will encounter a patient in hospital or under his or her care who has a spiritual need(s).

Activity 4.1

Before reading the rest of this chapter, spend a few moments reflecting upon your understanding of the 'nursing process'. Write down any thoughts or experiences that come to mind.

You may well have asked yourself what this exercise has to do with the provision of spiritual care. The answer is that an individual who is experiencing a spiritual need, as described in Chapter 2, may require such a need to be systematically addressed by the nurse. Once the need (problem) has been identified, or disclosed by the patient, a goal will need to be formulated. After a prescribed period of time an evaluation should be undertaken to establish whether the intervention or actions taken by the nurse (team) have been effective. This summary is an oversimplification and there are many issues surrounding spirituality and the nursing process that will be addressed during the rest of the chapter.

When undertaking Activity 4.1 several thoughts or experiences may have come to mind. First, you may have recalled that the nursing process is a way of organizing nursing care for patients using a problem-solving approach. Second, you may know that the nursing process is systematic and cyclical, involving a series of steps or stages starting with assessment and ending with an evaluation of the effectiveness of the care provided (Fig. 4.1).

The nursing process provides a 'safety' mechanism for assessment and evaluation of care. In recent years numerous types and variations of care plan have come into existence, for example core care plans (Cowell & Swiers 1997), critical or care pathways (Currie & Harvey 1998) and multidisciplinary collaborative care plans (Scott & Bowen 1997). Despite the emergence of these new methods of recording care, it can be argued that the principles of the nursing process still apply and are fundamental to their success.

Research undertaken by British nurse researchers (Waugh 1992, Narayanasamy 1993, McSherry 1998) indicates that nurses are encountering patients with spiritual needs during the course of their daily practice. Such research findings stress

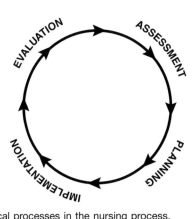

Figure 4.1   Cyclical processes in the nursing process.

Assessment: Conducting a spiritual assessment, recognizing a patient's spiritual need(s). It is important to be aware that assessment does not end after initial admission but that it is a continuous on-going process of observation and possible re-assessment.

Planning: The identification of those factors that are important to the individual's spirituality. This leads to the setting of goals, short- or long-term, that may be achievable by the individual in meeting his or her spiritual need.

Implementation: The identification and, where appropriate, the documentation of those interventions that may be instrumental in meeting the spiritual need(s) or enabling the patient to maintain his or her own spiritual needs while ill.

Evaluation: The identification of a criterion that may indicate that a patient's spiritual need(s) has been sufficiently addressed. The patient may report a sense of spiritual well-being or a feeling of being at peace with himself or herself or the situation.

In summary, the nursing process enables us as nurses to identify a patient's nursing problem(s) or needs, placing them in a systematic plan of care that is individualized and patient-centred, irrespective of the patient's underlying condition. The diagram illustrates the cyclical nature of spiritual assessment. We are continuously reassessing, implementing and re-evaluating care.

the importance of having some mechanism to ensure that patients' spiritual needs will be effectively addressed and met in clinical practice.

THE NURSING PROCESS

Kratz (1979 p. 3) states:

The nursing process is a problem-solving approach to nursing that involves interaction with the patient, making decisions and carrying out nursing actions based on an assessment of an individual patient's situation. It is followed by an evaluation of the effectiveness of our actions.

It is not unreasonable or unrealistic to apply this systematic approach to an individual who presents with a spiritual need. Ross (1996) suggests that spiritual care should be delivered to patients and taught to nurses within the framework of the nursing process. However, in recent times the nursing process has been the subject of much debate and criticism. Marks-Maran (1999) feels that it is now outdated. Despite recent criticism, the four stages involved in the nursing process – assessment, planning, implementation and evaluation (Fig. 4.1) – can still be applied to problems of a spiritual nature (Harrison & Burnard 1993). Each of these stages will be addressed in detail during the rest of the chapter. However, it must be emphasized that the main principles of the nursing process may need to be modified to meet an individual's circumstances. Spiritual problems do not fit neatly into each stage of the nursing process because these needs are usually complex. In fact spiritual needs may go unrecognized during an initial assessment (McSherry 1996). These issues will be explored through the use of case studies and reflective exercises.

Documentation

Another point that must be borne in mind when addressing the nursing process is the issue of documentation. The importance of documentation or record-keeping within health care has generated much debate in relation to legal and ethical issues (UKCC 1998). In stressing the importance of documentation a simple principle applies. If a nurse's, or indeed any health care professional's, care or actions are disputed, bringing into question the quality or standard of the care provided, then if nothing is written there will be nothing in the defence – a 'belt and braces mentality'. However, where a patient's problem originates from the spiritual dimension, owing to the sensitive and deeply personal nature of the issue identified, it may not be appropriate to document the concern or even devise a care plan. Patient confidentiality is a very important issue when providing spiritual care. These legal and ethical issues will be addressed towards the end of the chapter.

ASSESSMENT

The first stage in the nursing process is assessment of an individual's care needs. Assessment involves the gathering of information, perhaps from a wide range of sources, i.e. patient, medical records or family, by various means such as questioning or observation, in order to identify the patient's actual or potential problems. As you may recall, an assessment framework that is widely used in the UK involves the 12 activities of daily living based on or derived from the Roper, Logan & Tierney 'model of living', discussed in Chapter 3. These activities are used as a checklist or template to provide some structure for the admission assessment.

Activity 4.2   Admission exercise

Read Case study 4.1. Then write down on a piece of paper the types of questions that you might ask Mr Smith during the admission procedure.

Case study 4.1

Mr Smith, a 75-year-old retired miner, is admitted onto your ward with a chest infection. Mr Smith has been unwell for several weeks. He has become extremely breathless upon exertion and has developed a productive cough. He reports that he has recently been bereaved, his wife dying from breast cancer.

The admitting nurse might use the 12 activities of daily living as a mechanism for systematically enquiring into all aspects of the individual's life – in principle an individualized, patient-centred and holistic approach, providing a comprehensive and detailed assessment of the individual's normal function, and subsequent needs (Fig. 4.2). However, the assessment and identification of a patient's spiritual needs may be problematic. Because of the sensitive nature of spirituality, an individual may not share or reveal such information during an initial assessment since spirituality is normally incorporated under the section 'dying'. However, many care plans or admission records now incorporate a section entitled 'spiritual needs'.

Normal activity of daily living	Changes due to present illness/admission	Problem no.	Signature and date
Maintaining a safe environment			
Eating and drinking			
Breathing: Mr Smith smokes 30 cigarettes per day. He has no family history of breathing problems such as asthma or bronchitis.	Mr Smith reports that he has become very breathless upon the slightest of exertion. He has noticed a wheeze and says that he is coughing up thick green sputum.		
Elimination			
Communication			
Washing and dressing			
Mobilizing			
Temperature			
Dying	Mr Smith reports that he has recently been bereaved, as his wife died of breast cancer 6 months ago. He states that he has no fears about death, and that 'When you are dead, that's the end of everything.'		
Sleeping			
Working and recreation: Mr Smith worked as a miner for 35 years before being made redundant after the mines closed. He likes to have a game of darts, a couple of nights a week, at his local with his mates.	Mr Smith feels that he will miss his weekly visits to his local for a pint and a game of darts – 'Since my wife's death I like the company.'		
Expressing sexuality			
Spiritual needs: Mr Smith devoted a great deal of time caring for his wife who had terminal cancer. He does not believe in any life after death. He is adamant that there is no God and that religion is only trouble.	Mr Smith feels that since becoming ill he has started to question what life is all about. He finds it difficult to understand why some individuals seem to have more suffering and pain than others. He states that he does not want to see a chaplain.		

Figure 4.2 Admission assessment.

Undertaking this exercise may have been easy in relation to several of the categories that address physical activities, such as eating, drinking or breathing. However, there may have been some areas of Mr Smith's life that were difficult to assess such as his recent bereavement, his own attitudes towards death and dying, or even issues surrounding spiritual needs or sexuality. It has been recognized that there are several aspects of nursing that are considered taboo; these include sexuality, death and dying, and matters concerning spirituality. Nurses and other health care practitioners may overlook these areas when assessing a patient.

Activity 4.3

Reflecting upon your own clinical experience, can you recall the number of care plans that you have encountered that have addressed or identified in detail a patient's spirituality or spiritual needs?

Your reflections may reveal that you have encountered very few care plans or admission assessment forms that have identified a patient's spiritual need(s) while in hospital or out in the community. You may have recalled that in the 'spiritual needs' section the patient's religious beliefs had been written such as C of E (Church of England) or RC (Roman Catholic). You may also have identified that on many occasions the section was left blank or empty. There are several reasons for the box remaining blank; these are listed in Box 4.1.

In order to address the fears and apprehensions that nurses may experience when asked to address or assess matters of a

Box 4.1 Reasons for spiritual needs section being left empty

The subject of spiritual needs is felt too intrusive and personal to address on admission.
The admitting nurse did not feel comfortable in addressing such questions.
The patient did not want to answer the question or did not identify any spiritual needs at the time of admission.
The patient, and indeed the nurse, did not understand the term 'spiritual needs'.
The patient identified a spiritual need that was felt too private and sensitive to write or disclose in his or her care plan.

spiritual nature, several authors have devised questions or guidelines that may make spiritual assessment easier.

Stoll (1979) presents some guidelines for undertaking a spiritual assessment.

Concept of God or deity. The types of questions that may be asked by the nurse addressing this aspect of spirituality are: Is religion or God significant to you? If yes, can you describe how? Is prayer helpful to you? What happens when you pray? (Stoll 1979 p. 1572).

Sources of hope and strength. Who is the most important person to you? To whom do you turn when you need help? Are they available (Stoll 1979 p. 1575).

Religious practices. Do you feel that your faith (or religion) is helpful to you? If yes, would you tell me how? Are there any religious practices that are important to you?

Relationship between spiritual beliefs and health. What has bothered you most about being sick (or in what is happening to you)? What do you think is going to happen to you?

Activity 4.4

Spend several minutes reflecting upon these guidelines and write down your first impressions.

It is suggested that assessment in relation to the identification of spiritual needs must be an 'ongoing' exercise. Questioning an individual about his or her religious orientation or spiritual needs may be appropriate and helpful, on admission to hospital or when first meeting them in the community, in identifying those individuals for whom religious affiliation and practice are fundamental to their spiritual well-being. However, caution must be exercised as for the unbeliever, atheists or agnostic (Burnard 1988) this type of questioning may be threatening. Stoll's guidelines do suggest the types of areas that may need to be addressed within a spiritual assessment. She herself, towards the end of her article (Stoll 1979 p. 1577), writes:

Neither sexual nor spiritual values should be introduced at the beginning of the interview. I have found it beneficial to separate sexuality from spiritual concerns with questions pertaining to physical

Caution

There is a danger in making spiritual assessment mechanistic, reducing it to a tick box exercise that may negate the use of other modes of continuous assessment (Catterall et al 1998). This can be illustrated by the following question: What if a patient is assessed by one nurse on admission who felt that the patient did not, at the time of admission, have any spiritual needs. Does this mean that such an individual may not develop a spiritual need(s) during the course of their illness or hospitalization? If you can recall Murray & Zentner's (1989) definition, this seems to support the principle of continuous assessment since during their period of illness or hospitalization individuals may begin to question the meaning of life or the implications of illness (Simsen 1985), perhaps facing the prospect of death. Such existential questions may not be raised, or identified, when a patient is first admitted into hospital.

The dangers or problems that can arise when even the most basic of spiritual assessments is not undertaken during admission to hospital are raised in Case study 4.2.

and social needs. The spiritual dimension lends itself to being a continuation of the psychosocial assessment toward the latter part of an interview.

This quotation highlights the sensitivity that has to be employed when discussing spiritual concerns. Two major questions must be considered before nurses, chaplains and

Case study 4.2   Spiritual care: a case to answer

Peter, 72 years old, was known by his family and friends to like a short or two. He was admitted to hospital with an acute episode of chest pain. A diagnosis of angina was made since ECGs showed no evidence of recent infarct.

It came to light later that Peter was a practising Roman Catholic who found meaning and purpose in his beliefs. Peter had only been in hospital overnight and he had not seen his wife because she had taken herself off to their daughters 'down south' after an argument. Nevertheless she was informed by Peter of his admission into hospital and she was intending to visit as soon as possible. In the afternoon on the following day Peter was due to be discharged when he developed sudden severe central chest pain, collapsing with a cardiac arrest – resuscitation was initiated. During the resuscitation Peter's wife arrived on the ward. Unfortunately she did not see Peter before he died. After Peter's death his wife asked if the Catholic priest had been. Inspection of the nursing notes showed that nothing in relation to religion had been entered.

academics 'steam roll' ahead in designing complex assessment criteria:

Can spiritual needs be identified by the use of assessment tools? For example those used to predict or identify those individuals at risk of developing a pressure sore, i.e. Waterlow score?

Can spiritual needs be predicted by such mechanistic interventions and calculations? The definitions of spirituality presented in Chapter 2 demonstrate that it is a very subjective, complex and individually determined aspect of life.

Activity 4.5

Having read the case study surrounding Peter, can you identify any issues that you feel it generates in relation to the assessment of an individual's spiritual needs?

In response to this question you may have identified that there is an important need for a brief assessment of an individual's religious orientation and practices. In Peter's case his religious beliefs were a fundamental part of his spirituality. His Catholic faith had become interwoven into his beliefs and all dimensions of his life. By omitting to identify Peter's religious practices the nurses had failed in their duty to provide 'holistic' care. The case study stresses the role of the nurse in documenting even the simplest of information. We are all probably guilty of skipping the question surrounding religion, as demonstrated when reflecting upon your own practice earlier. Peter's case highlights the important role that nurses play in communicating, maintaining and identifying a patient's religious practices to others in the multidisciplinary team such as the hospital chaplains or the patient's own religious leader. A failure to undertake the crudest of spiritual assessments, which may initially only ask about a patient's religious beliefs and practices, can prove detrimental to the patient. It could be argued that Peter's case is extreme, but nevertheless it highlights the important point that there is no room for complacency when addressing matters of spirituality.

The case study demonstrates how failure to provide spiritual care may influence the attitudes of patients and their next of kin about the standard and quality of care being provided. One cannot read Peter's case without thinking that the nursing profession had failed his wife. She had witnessed care that was fragmented and not individual because it was ineffectual in that it did not recognize her husband's spirituality.

It has been suggested in this section that assessment of spiritual needs should be ongoing and continuous. There are several methods or measures that can be used that assist in identifying a patient(s) who has a spiritual need(s) (adapted from Carson 1989 p. 158).

Direct questioning. We have demonstrated that this may be inappropriate, threatening and perceived as intrusive. However, it may be used to elicit information quickly about religious beliefs and practices upon admission.

Observation of non-verbal and verbal behaviour. The individual may be withdrawn or look and act frustrated or agitated. His or her body language may suggest that the person is depressed. The person may physically seek solitude or isolation (McSherry 1996). Does the person pray or use other symbolic gestures? However, it must be stressed that these types of behaviour may also be indicative of concern that is not related to a spiritual need but still requires addressing. With reference to the verbal behaviours that may indicate that a person has a spiritual need, you may notice that the individual is always complaining out of all proportion. He or she may call upon God in a derogatory way. During the course of a conversation the patient may question the meaning of his or her health problem, life or future prognosis. These forms of verbal behaviour may indicate that an individual is having difficulty accepting or reconciling some issue that is affecting his or her very existence, or they may be indicative of an issue that is nothing to do with the person's spirituality.

Interpersonal. Most patient have visitors or family and friends. However, there may be occasions when a patient does not have anyone visiting. This may indicate that a person is living alone and perhaps is isolated – a point worth clarifying with the person. Some patients may have representatives of their faith visiting frequently, indicating their belief and involvement in a particular faith. On odd occasions after a patient has had visitors he or she may appear frustrated,

---

Case study 4.3

An elderly man had been admitted onto the ward several days earlier for medical observation and assessment for bowel problems. In the night he required an emergency operation. When gathering together the patient's belongings to transfer them across to the surgical ward while the patient was in theatre, nurses came across an old Bible with dog-eared pages. This revealed the patient's personal belief in a God. It also alerted nurses to the fact that the man did have a personal spiritual belief that nurses could help him meet. The man had been too ill to disclose his beliefs on admission and he had no family or friends to ask.

---

angered or annoyed, indicating that their relationships are not entirely harmonious or supportive.

Environmental. The patient might wear a religious artefact, such as a medal or a cross. Their cards may be of a religious nature. They may read religious material or holy books such as the Bible. The example above illustrates the importance of observational assessment (see Case study 4.3).

PLANNING

After assessment there is a need to use the information gained to formulate a plan of care. Where possible this should be done in collaboration with the patient. The information should be collated and verified with the patient and then goal(s) should be set that are realistic, patient-centred, and in a time frame that is acceptable to the patient and the nurse. Planning is probably the most difficult aspect of using a problem-solving approach. With reference to a physical problem such as nausea and vomiting or relieving the discomfort associated with a high temperature, the plan or goal can usually be drawn up easily. For example Mrs Jones will report that her nausea has been relieved within 30 minutes of it developing. The formulation of such goals is not so easy with problems arising from a spiritual need(s).

Activity 4.6   Planning care

Reread Case study 2.2 and the subsequent section addressing Jim's spiritual needs (the case study is reproduced here as Case study 4.4). Now devise a plan of care that you feel would enable Jim to meet the spiritual need shown by his loss of meaning, purpose and fulfilment.

Case study 4.4   Time to think

Jim, 65 years old, was admitted to the ward with a grossly swollen right leg, thigh and calf. A diagnosis of DVT (deep vein thrombosis) was made. He was started on a heparin infusion and kept on total bed rest because of the severe pain when he mobilized.

One morning while the nurse was talking to Jim he became very emotional and began to cry. As the nurse listened to him it emerged that on 24 December it was the first anniversary of his wife's death. Jim recalled how he had been married for 45 years and for the last 10 years of his married life had been the main carer for his wife, who suffered from rheumatoid arthritis. Jim went on to describe how lonely and depressed he felt, stating that a day did not pass without him thinking about his wife and the wonderful life they had shared together. Jim is not a religious man but he does believe in life after death.

Having read the case study you have probably identified that Jim has several different spiritual needs that need to be addressed, such as the need for meaning and purpose, the need for trust, and a need for a loving relationship. You may also have found it difficult to articulate or write a goal. The overall result may be one of frustration, leaving only a series of questions:

How do you go about setting goals and establishing a criterion against which spiritual needs can be measured?
How do you determine whether a goal can be met in the short or long term?
Are there not some ethical issues about writing down something that is deeply personal and private?
How can you write a goal for needs that seem so subjective and complex?

The writing of care plans is often very difficult and time consuming. It could be argued that one reason for having core care plans or critical pathways is to reduce the amount of time that qualified nurses spend on completing paperwork. Time spent with paperwork could mean less time spent with the patient. However, such sentiments would not stand up in a court of law – remember, if there is nothing written, then there is nothing in your defence. Core care plans or critical pathways do not really accommodate the subjective and complex nature of spiritual needs because such needs are so unique and individually determined that they do not lend themselves to flow charts or tick box exercises. Therefore if a patient's spiritual needs are to be addressed in a plan of care, then usually the nurse will have to work through the stages in the nursing process. A goal needs to be formulated and time limits for evaluation set, with the planning taking place in conjunction with the patient.

GOALS

Setting goals that can address spiritual needs requires flexibility and sensitivity. Goals should be grounded in reality – they should be achievable. A problem with some spiritual needs is that they cannot be resolved in the short term. For example in Case study 4.4 Jim had lost meaning and purpose in his life after the death of his wife. It would be totally unrealistic to expect the goals for his spiritual care to be met overnight (see Box 4.2). There are many issues that Jim will have to face and explore before his life has new meaning and purpose. It is the lack of concrete solutions and quick fixes that makes the setting of goals difficult when trying to address a patient's spiritual need(s). It is very likely that it will take Jim many months before he has totally come to terms with the death of his wife and resolved the loss and spiritual pain that he experienced. Having stated this, it is not unrealistic to start a

---

Box 4.2 Jim's plan of care

Identified patient concern/problem
Jim has identified that he has lost all meaning and purpose in life, and that he feels lonely and depressed since his wife's death.

Goal
While in hospital the goal is to enable Jim to evaluate his life in order to rediscover value, meaning and purpose.

Plan of care
The nurses should allow time for Jim to explore and discuss the fears and worries that have destroyed meaning and value in his life.

All members of staff should treat Jim with dignity and respect, fostering a relationship of trust – perhaps restoring confidence and hope.

The nurse should identify with Jim the areas in his life that he may find enjoyable and meaningful, using these as a platform on which to build self-esteem.

If it was felt appropriate, Jim could refer himself to an external agency that would be able to provide support and counselling upon discharge.

---

patient on the journey of reflection and acceptance while in hospital or under the care of a health professional.

IMPLEMENTATION

Implementing a plan of care means that energy and time are being committed to reaching a desired goal or outcome that has been set by the patient in conjunction with the nurse. With reference to the meeting of a spiritual need, the plan usually involves an element of time on the nurse's part spent actively listening to the patient's concerns. Time may also be spent liaising with others in the multidisciplinary team, for example informing or arranging a visit by the hospital chaplain or the patient's own religious or spiritual leader. The plan of care may also see the nurse organizing the environment in order to allow the patient time alone and privacy in which to pray or reflect. The plan of care will ultimately be determined by whatever spiritual need(s) a patient presents with. A patient whose spiritual need(s) are based on maintaining their spiritual practices may be accommodated by allowing time for the patient to pray or read in private. It may entail organizing care and staff so that the patient can attend a communion service in the chapel on Sunday or a holy day of obligation. It may mean contacting the patient's religious or spiritual leaders and notifying them that they have been admitted into hospital or that an individual has died so that specific rites and rituals can be performed in accordance with the person's religious customs. This reinforces the need to obtain as much detail and information about a person's religious practices upon admission so that insight can be gained and appropriate actions implemented.

The critical incident analysis in Case study 4.5 demonstrates how detailed assessment influences all the different stages in the nursing process – planning, implementation, right through to evaluation. Effective spiritual care cannot be offered to a patient(s) unless sufficient information has been obtained during assessment (continuous) and communicated to all staff involved in care delivery – from consultant to housekeeper. A plan of care that highlights what an individual's spiritual need(s) are and how these needs are to be met allows everyone to work together to achieve the desired goal. Spiritual care, indeed all types of care, will be fragmented and goals will not be effectively reached if everyone is working in isolation and implementing their own plan of care. You may recall how frustrating it can be when you have applied a particular wound dressing for a patient, writing instructions in the care plan. Returning on duty the next day you find that one of your colleagues has ignored your plan of care and applied something different from what you documented. Continuity is lost and everyone, including the patient, is left feeling confused. This illustration also highlights issues of accountability.

Case study 4.5 Critical incident analysis

A patient had not really eaten a substantial meal since being admitted into hospital two days previously. The patient in question had suffered a stroke several years earlier that had left him with expression dysphasia. Investigating the matter, it emerged that the patient was a vegan and since admission had been given meat or dairy products at meal times. With insight it was obvious why the patient had refused to eat, as he had been offended by the diet offered. This critical incident analysis highlights the value and importance individuals attach to their own personal, cultural beliefs and practices. It also reinforces the need for a systematic way of communicating and implementing patient care.

EVALUATION

It could be said that evaluation is the final stage of the nursing process, and possibly the most difficult to undertake in relation to establishing whether an individual's spiritual need(s) have been met. Nursing interventions that seek to address physical problems are usually easier to review. For example making tracings or taking photographs of a patient's leg ulcer upon admission or before commencing a treatment regime would provide a baseline for subsequent evaluation. Three weeks later the ulcer is retraced or new photographs taken. Comparisons with the drawings or photographs will reveal any improvement or deterioration, indicating whether the care is effective or the desired goal achieved.

The same principle can be applied to an individual whose spiritual needs have their origin within a religious framework. It is easy to establish whether these types of spiritual need have been met by ensuring the patient attends a particular service or documenting that their religious/spiritual leader has been to visit. However, things are not so 'black and white' when trying to evaluate spiritual needs that are very subjective, involving the ordinary and mundane aspects of life. As you will recall, spiritual needs are uniquely determined by the individual. The problems arise because there is no baseline or criterion against which future comparisons can be made and progress determined, for example how does the nurse set about reviewing or evaluating whether a person is starting to regain meaning and purpose in life? Or how does one determine whether a person feels reconciled or forgiven? These two questions indicate the problematic nature of evaluating whether a patient's spiritual needs have been met.

Consultation and participation are the two key ingredients in determining the effectiveness of spiritual interventions. The patient should be consulted and asked to comment upon how he or she feels that progress is being made towards meeting a specific spiritual need. The patient might reveal that he or she is feeling more optimistic about the future. Another indicator that a spiritual need is being addressed may be found in how an individual describes himself or herself. Words like relaxed, at peace, or inner calm may indicate a refocusing of spirituality. Earlier the importance of observation as a means of assessment was discussed. As with assessment, observation can be used as an aid to evaluation. The nurse may observe for verbal and non-verbal behaviours that may indicate a change in attitude or inner disposition. An individual who was extremely withdrawn may display behaviour that suggests a more relaxed openness towards staff or other patients – communicating more freely.

Difficulties

Another problem with evaluation is the setting of realistic time limits for review. As stated earlier, it may take an individual many months to come to terms with a health problem or personal crisis that has brought into question his or her entire existence. It would be unrealistic to expect such an individual to reflect, adjust and regain composure in a matter of hours, days or possibly weeks. Therefore setting realistic dates for the review of a spiritual need must take into consideration the individual and the spiritual need that has been identified or disclosed. To say that it will take three days for a patient to establish trust and one week for an individual to regain meaning and purpose in his or her life after a diagnosis of Type II diabetes mellitus would be very prescriptive. This type of approach would be totally unrealistic and ineffective, contradicting everything that has been discussed in this chapter. Therefore evaluation of spiritual needs requires sensitivity and common sense in that there needs to be a realization on the nurse's part that individuals will meet their own spiritual needs at a pace determined by the patients themselves.

This section has highlighted the difficulties associated with evaluation of spiritual needs, especially those needs that are very subjective. Having stated this, evaluation needs to be undertaken in order to assess an individual's progress, identifying any measures that the nurse can implement to assist in the goal being met. If problems are encountered then the goal may need to be reassessed and an alternative strategy devised and implemented.

ETHICAL CONSIDERATIONS

Throughout this chapter you may be pausing and reflecting upon the material, asking yourself several fundamental questions around assessment, documentation, continuity of care, accountability and confidentiality.

Activity 4.7

Read Case study 4.6 and identify any ethical issues that you feel are apparent or applicable to this case.

Case study 4.6 is complex, addressing several important aspects of spirituality such as the need for inner peace (McSherry 1996). The case study reinforces how spirituality is related to all aspects of a person's being. Reading the case study you may have identified that there are several important ethical issues raised, such as confidentiality, accountability and advocacy. These ethical issues bring into question many of the

---

Case study 4.6   The need for a team approach

Pamela, 27 years old, was admitted to the ward with a recent history of weight loss and anorexia. On admission she looked very pale and thin and had a body mass index of 19, indicating that she was possibly malnourished. The medical team could find no physical or pathological explanation to account for her condition.

Pamela was a highly anxious individual who had been suffering from anxiety and depression for several months. Therefore the medical team concluded that her anorexia and weight loss were associated with her high anxiety state. She was seen by a dietician and referred to a psychiatrist.

Pamela had a great deal of support and understanding from her partner, with whom she had three children. During the course of her hospitalization she became very emotional and frustrated at the medical staff's inability to find any physical explanation for her condition. On one occasion she ran off following a procedure that did not discover any pathology and was found sitting outside, crying bitterly. After being encouraged and supported back to the day room, Pamela revealed to the nurse that she had had a termination of pregnancy earlier that year, which she now felt ashamed and embarrassed about. She recalled how at that time her partner was out of work, having been made redundant, and they felt that financially it would be unfair to bring another child into their family.

Owing to numerous interruptions in the day room the nurse felt that it would be unfair to continue with the conversation and that they should resume at another time. Pamela did state that she had always been an anxious individual, but her anxiety and depression had increased soon after this event; she asked the nurse not to mention this to anyone. The following day the nurse arrived back on duty to find that Pamela had been discharged home that morning with an outpatient appointment to see the psychiatrist and dietician.

---

principles surrounding the use of the nursing process or documentation as a framework for providing spiritual care.

Continuity of care

In the case study the nurse was starting to address a spiritual need, only to find that the patient had been discharged. Pamela's situation highlights the difficulties that patients and nurses may encounter when disclosing and addressing spiritual concerns. The circumstances in the case study reveal how continuity of care can be problematic. This raises a question: How ethical is it to start to address a patient's spiritual pain – possibly 'opening a can of worms' – to find that there is no means of closure or developing a relationship that may be therapeutic?

The fast throughput of patients in acute and critical care settings may mean that the continuity of care that is vital if patients' spiritual needs are to be effectively met can be limited. Pamela's case underlines the need for a team approach in the meeting of patients' spiritual needs. It is no good just the nurses being spiritually aware. This awareness and sensitivity towards problems of a spiritual nature needs to be adopted by medical and other professions allied to medicine. If this awareness is not universally shared then spiritual needs in patients will always go unrecognized or dismissed as undeserving of medical attention or intervention. In some instances a referral to the psychiatrist or hospital chaplain may be counter-productive.

Discharge policy

Another important issue in relation to continuity is discharge planning and referrals. It has been indicated that spiritual needs that are complex, involving matters addressing meaning, purpose and fulfilment in life, may not be resolved in the short term. Is it ethical and reasonable to expect nurses or chaplains to provide support to individuals with such needs while in hospital, if they are to be discharged with the individual's spiritual concerns only partially addressed? This point brings into question issues about continuity of care between acute and community, primary care settings. Interestingly, the National Health Service Executive (Northern and Yorkshire regions) in 1995 devised 'a framework for spiritual faith and pastoral related care'. Close inspection of this document does not give any acknowledgement to this problem. Neither does the framework make any suggestions as to how solutions to this ethical dilemma may be formulated. It would appear that there is an urgent need to develop a national standard that addresses these problems of continuity of care.

Documentation (revisited)

Throughout this chapter the importance of documentation has been emphasized. However, Pamela's case study demonstrates the personal and sensitive nature of spiritual needs. Would it have been right to have written something so personal and confidential in a plan of care, with the potential for everyone to read it? Another area of concern would be if Pamela had asked specifically for all the information she had entrusted to the nurse to remain private and confidential – neither wanting anything written nor anything verbally disclosed. This type of request can be very challenging and threatening because the nurse is torn 'between the devil and the deep blue sea'. The dilemma is that if you do not disclose or document something, then an event may occur that could have been prevented if others had been fully informed. However, there are no easy ethical solutions and the result is often to be found in collaboration and communication within a safe and confidential relationship between the patient and the nurse in whom the patient has confided.

Confidentiality

Pamela's case study highlights the deeply personal and sensitive nature of spirituality. It demonstrates clearly how situations and circumstance in life can change, bringing into question motives and moral decision-making and reasoning. However, would it be right for the nurse to have disclosed such personal facts to other staff? Should such personal situations be documented in a plan of care? These are very important questions that nurses must ask when addressing matters of a spiritual nature. Patients may feel more secure if they know that a problem that they have divulged to you is safe. You are probably well aware that any breach of confidentiality, however small, can destroy the patient's trust, and all measures being taken to help meet a patient's spiritual needs will be futile. Such dilemmas put the nurse in a very precarious situation, a little like the priest in a confessional who receives some information that could save lives but the details cannot be disclosed because of the seal of confession. To say that there are easy solutions to such dilemmas would be very prescriptive and unrealistic. Many of these situations are dependent upon individual circumstances and usually solutions are to be found in the situation itself. An example of this is that often after some time reflecting the patient may acknowledge that there is a need for further help and ask for the information to be passed on to the appropriate professionals or agencies. However, this does not remove or diminish the level of responsibility or pressure that a nurse may experience when he or she is privy to confidential matters concerning a patient. At times being responsible for such information can leave individual nurses feeling under pressure and both emotionally challenged and isolated.

Advocacy

This implies that nurses should act in a manner that will promote and safeguard the interests and well-being of patients or clients within the sphere of their care (UKCC 1992). The principle of advocacy is often difficult and problematic to apply in practice. This is evident in Pamela's situation. In order to address Pamela's spiritual needs, maintain trust and confidence, the nurse is obliged not to disclose the spiritual matters that have resulted in her loss of spiritual well-being. On the other hand the nurse is aware that if the spiritual needs are documented and disclosed, then this would inform the course of her care and subsequent decisions made by the medical and nursing team.

CONCLUSION

This chapter has explored how spiritual care can be provided within the framework of the nursing process of assessment, planning, implementation and evaluation. Through the use of case studies spiritual needs that may arise within clinical practice have been presented. Implicitly it is acknowledged that the entire area of care planning and documentation are fundamental in the delivery of the highest quality nursing care. This principle is also relevant when addressing patients whose problems have their origin within the spiritual realm. The information provided addressing spirituality and the nursing process is not prescriptive, acknowledging that there are no easy solutions to be found to often-complex ethical dilemmas. The chapter has continued the need for reflection upon practice in order to develop insight and new knowledge.

REFERENCES

Burnard P 1988 The spiritual needs of atheists and agnostics. Professional Nurse December: 130–132
Carson V B 1989 Spiritual dimensions of nursing practice. W B Saunders, Philadelphia, ch 7, pp 150–179

Catteral R A, Cox M, Greet B, Sankey J, Griffiths G 1998 The assessment and audit of spiritual care. International Journal of Palliative Nursing 4 (4): 162–168

Cowell J, Swiers D 1997 Trust-wide core care plans. Nursing Standard 12 (4): 39–41

Currie L, Harvey G 1998 Care pathways development and implementation. Nursing Standard 12 (30): 35–38

Harrison J, Burnard P 1993 Spirituality and nursing practice. Avebury, Aldershot

Kratz C R 1979 The nursing process. Baillière Tindall, London

McSherry W 1996 Raising the spirits. Nursing Times 92 (3): 48–49

McSherry W 1998 Nurses' perceptions of spirituality and spiritual care. Nursing Standard 13 (4): 36–40

Marks-Maran D 1999 Reconstructing nursing: evidence, artistry and curriculum. Nurse Education Today 19: 3–10

Murray R B, Zentner J B 1989 Nursing concepts for health promotion. Prentice Hall, London

Narayanasamy A 1993 Nurses' awareness and educational preparation in meeting their patients' spiritual needs. Nurse Education Today 13 (3): 196–201

Narayanasamy A 1996 Spiritual care of chronically ill patients. British Journal of Nursing 5 (7): 411–416

Ross L 1996 Teaching spiritual care to nurses. Nurse Education Today 16: 38–43

Scott E, Bowen B 1997 Multidisciplinary collaborative care planning. Nursing Standard 12 (1): 39–42

Simsen B 1985 Spiritual needs and resources in illness and hospitalisation. Unpublished MSc thesis, University of Manchester, Manchester

Stoll R 1979 Guidelines for spiritual assessment. American Journal of Nursing 79: 1574–1577

United Kingdom Central Council for Nursing, Midwifery and Health Visiting 1992 Code of professional conduct. UKCC, London

United Kingdom Central Council for Nursing, Midwifery and Health Visiting 1998 Guidelines for record keeping. UKCC, London

Waugh L 1992 Spiritual aspects of nursing: a descriptive study of nurses' perceptions. Unpublished PhD thesis, Queen Margaret College, Edinburgh

FURTHER READING

These texts will develop your insight into the issues surrounding the provision of spiritual care. They will clarify how spiritual needs can be addressed with the framework of the nursing process.

Burnard P 1988 The spiritual needs of atheists and agnostics. Professional Nurse December: 130–132

Carson V B 1989 Spiritual dimensions of nursing practice. W B Saunders, Philadelphia, ch 7, pp 150–179

Catteral R A, Cox M, Greet B, Sankey J, Griffiths G 1998 The assessment and audit of spiritual care. International Journal of Palliative Nursing 4 (4): 162–168

Harrison J, Burnard P 1993 Spirituality and nursing practice. Avebury, Aldershot

McSherry W 1996 Raising the spirits. Nursing Times 92 (3): 48–49

Ross L A 1994 Spiritual aspects of nursing. Journal of Advanced Nursing 19: 439–447

Ross L 1997 The nurse's role in assessing and responding to patients' spiritual needs. International Journal of Palliative Nursing 3 (1): 37–42

Stoll R 1979 Guidelines for spiritual assessment. American Journal of Nursing 79: 1574–1577

5

Barriers influencing the provision of spiritual care

INTRODUCTION

This chapter focuses upon the intrinsic barriers (within the individual) and extrinsic barriers (within the health care situation) that affect nurses' ability to provide spiritual care. The chapter will explore in detail the barriers that exist in practice, presenting some strategies and solutions that may empower nurses better to meet an individual's spiritual needs. Case studies are used to generate a deeper awareness and insight into the barriers identified that result in spiritual needs remaining unmet.

Activity 5.1

Using material explored earlier in this book, can you identify any barriers that may prevent nurses from addressing or meeting their patients' spiritual needs?

Box 5.1   The two main categories of barriers

Intrinsic
   The word intrinsic is used in this context to mean any factor arising
   within an individual that may affect the provision of spiritual care.
Extrinsic
   The word extrinsic is used to describe factors that arise beyond the
   control of an individual, which prevent or inhibit the provision of
   spiritual care.

Having reflected upon the case studies presented in earlier chapters you may have identified several points such as a lack of privacy, fear or ignorance. On closer inspection of your list you may note that the barriers can be placed into different categories: those that arise from within the nurse or patient; those concerned with communication; and a further selection that appear on initial reflection to be beyond the control of the nurse or patient. These barriers will now be explored in greater detail (Box 5.1).

IDENTIFYING THE BARRIERS

The growing realization that nurses can play a fundamental role in the provision of spiritual care has witnessed a proliferation in the amount of published material discussing this issue (Soeken & Carson 1987, Waugh 1992, Taylor et al 1994, McSherry 1998). As the 'caution' indicates, nursing could be accused of being overprescriptive in its approach to spiritual care if it does not exercise sensitivity and flexibility. It is all too easy to legislate for a particular action or manner of conduct without having an appreciation of the full picture. This point is highlighted by a line that appears in the discussion section of an article by Johnston et al (1994 p. 485):

Caution

When reviewing the literature concerning the nurse's ability to provide spiritual care, the nursing profession is at risk of being dogmatic. Many articles being published suggest that nurses should be providing spiritual care irrespective of patients' wishes. This tendency towards being overprescriptive must be considered when examining the barriers that may prevent nurses from providing spiritual care, because such dogmatism may be unjustified.

However, the somewhat moderate responses to the Likert items indicated these nurses' commitment to, or confidence about, spiritual care is not as strong as could be.

This quotation appears judgemental and extremely prescriptive, critical of nurses' practice in relation to their ability and confidence in meeting patients' spiritual needs. However, Soeken & Carson (1987 p. 610) write:

Meeting the spiritual needs of patients can be uncomfortable for the nurse. Several reasons for such discomforts include embarrassment, the belief that it is not the nurse's role, lack of training, and lack of own spiritual resources.

This quotation seems more balanced, emphasizing that the provision of spiritual care is not simple and straightforward because there are many factors that must be considered. A comparison of Soeken & Carson's quotation with your own list of barriers may reveal similarities.

Research undertaken by nurses in the UK has revealed barriers similar to those that exist in the USA. Ross (1994, 1997) identified that barriers could be nurse or patient related, profession related, or environmentally related. McSherry (1997) highlighted barriers similar in nature, describing them as economic, educational, environmental or personal in origin.

ACHIEVING POSITIVE SPIRITUAL CARE

Figure 5.1 illustrates how the successful provision of spiritual care is dependent upon three key areas – the nurse, the patient, and the economic and environmental context in which spiritual care is provided. It is suggested that for spiritual care to be effective all these three areas must be working in relative harmony. Barriers manifesting themselves in any of these areas will result in the patient's spiritual needs not necessarily being met as perceived by the patient. Intrinsic and extrinsic barriers to providing spiritual care will be discussed in more detail below.

INTRINSIC BARRIERS

I would probably rather tell you about my sex life than about my spiritual life. And I'm fairly sure you would be more scandalized to find a Bible at the bottom of my briefcase than a copy of the *Karma Sutra*. (Allen 1991 p. 52)

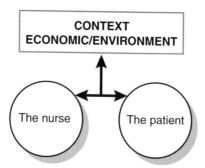

Figure 5.1 The three areas in which barriers may occur.

Charlotte Allen's quotation highlights the deeply personal aspects of spirituality, indicating that there are many personal barriers (intrinsic) that prevent us from addressing this dimension of care with individuals. It would seem that in today's society individuals feel more comfortable talking about sexuality and elimination than about spiritual matters. Implicit in the quotation is the notion that barriers in the provision of spiritual care may not only originate from within the patient, but also from within the nurse. The provision of spiritual care is an exchange of energy – an encounter – between two individuals: the nurse and patient, the doctor and the patient, or the patient and his or her own spiritual leader. Therefore barriers in the exchange of this energy may arise from within any of these key individuals.

The intrinsic barriers that may prevent the provision of spiritual care are not specific to the patient. Figure 5.1 shows that the provision of spiritual care is a two-way process between the patient and the nurse (Clark et al 1991). Therefore an

---

Box 5.2 Intrinsic barriers

Inability to communicate through illness or loss of senses
Ambiguity
Lack of knowledge in the area of spirituality
  Patient not aware of the concept of spiritual need
Sensitive area – too personal for nurses to address
  Own personal beliefs and values
Emotionally demanding and fear-provoking
  Fears – mismanagement
  Prejudices

intrinsic barrier may develop within either the nurse or the patient, preventing spiritual needs from being addressed. Some of the intrinsic barriers that may arise are listed in Box 5.2. Nurse researchers have identified several of these barriers (Waugh 1992, McSherry 1997).

Intrinsic barriers may be associated with our own personal belief systems, which may be in conflict with that of the patient. For example our attitudes towards certain religious groups may be prejudiced by the beliefs and values we have acquired through socialization. Another example may be the attitudes we have towards different sections in society, such as the social stigma attached to HIV and AIDS. Other barriers may occur as a result of our inability to communicate effectively with patients.

The barriers listed in Box 5.2 are discussed in detail below.

Inability to communicate through illness or loss of senses

McCavery (1985 p. 130) stresses the importance of good communication in providing spiritual care:

In many ways, spiritual care is subjective, and its success rests upon the meaning of conversations between individual patients and nurse.

Working from this quotation, a major obstacle in the provision of spiritual care is a breakdown in the channels of communication. Ross (1994) presents several conditions that can impede communication such as aphasia (loss of speech), or any other problem associated with the loss of a sense such as sight or hearing (see Case study 5.2). The inability to communicate effectively can result in an individual being unable to express a spiritual need, and the nurse being unable to assess or interpret the situation. The overall results of such situations may see the patient's spiritual needs remaining unrecognized and consequently unmet. This inability to communicate effectively can mean the patient and nurse become frustrated. Such situations are not easy to resolve, as there are no easy solutions. The nurse may use a variety of techniques to try and establish what the individual needs such as writing down needs, using word charts, or even enlisting an interpreter to translate a patient's needs.

Case study 5.1 How to proceed

Samantha is 8 years of age and diagnosed with an inoperable terminal brain tumour. Samantha has been told about her condition and seems to avoid any mention of the issue. She keeps repeating time and again, 'I do not want to die mammy'.
 What do you feel are the intrinsic issues that may be barriers in providing adequate spiritual care?

Another aspect of communication that can prove problematic is communicating effectively with individuals who may not have the intellectual development or intellectual capacity to think abstractly, such as young children or individuals with severe learning disabilities or clients with organic brain disease such as dementia (Case study 5.1).

This case study stresses the importance of providing spiritual care that is appropriate and at the correct level for individuals to comprehend. Sommer (1989 p. 231) highlights some of the difficulties practitioners may face when attending to the spiritual needs of dying children.

Children can readily sense when adults are uncomfortable with a topic of discussion or a situation. Whereas healthy children like to express their uniqueness, sick and dying children like to find ways of blending in with the crowd.

The issues identified in this quotation are certainly evident in Samantha's situation. The importance of good communication and interpersonal skills in managing such situations is paramount. If barriers exist that prevent channels of communication, then our human condition may result in avoidance of the situation. Samantha's situation is difficult with the potential for it to be emotionally demanding and exhausting. Such situations challenge and drain the emotional and spiritual reserves of the most experienced practitioners.

Ambiguity

Ambiguity is when uncertainty or a lack of insight into situations prevents either the nurse or the patient from entering into a therapeutic relationship. Numerous reasons for this may exist and it is not unique to the spiritual dimension. However, because of the deeply personal nature of spirituality ambiguity may arise when the nurse and patient have contrasting belief systems and personalities. This can be illustrated by the situation where a nurse who does not have any belief in God is asked to be primary nurse for a patient who is a practising Christian attending a very Evangelical church. At every opportunity the patient tries to convert the nurse. This situation may arouse a great deal of insecurity, frustration, and vulnerability within the nurse. The result may be that the nurse feels that his or her personal belief system is being challenged and where possible the nurse may avoid making any meaningful contact with the patient. Similarly a nurse may have strong beliefs about the sanctity of life and they may decline to participate in the surgical procedure of termination of pregnancy.

Lack of knowledge in the area of spirituality

Ambiguity may also arise when the patient or nurse does not know what is meant by the term 'spiritual need'. There is an urgent need for nursing to research more fully patients' and nurses' understanding of these terms. For ambiguity to be removed nurses need to be introspective, being aware of their own personal beliefs, values and, importantly, prejudices. Reflecting upon practice or critical incidents that are encountered in relation to spiritual matters will enable practitioners to evaluate their own emotions and feelings, formulating strategies that will allow them perhaps to cope better or adjust their practice should similar situations be encountered in the future (McSherry 1996).

Sensitive area – too personal for nurses to address

McSherry (1997) asked nurses to provide some qualitative responses into what they perceived were the main barriers in the provision of spiritual care. Several of the nurses surveyed indicated that the area of spirituality was too sensitive to be addressed by nurses. The notion of sensitivity included nurses' personal fears of mismanagement of personal situations. Harrison (1993) highlighted a particular concern related to over involvement in situations one cannot handle – 'getting out of one's depth'. Another aspect of sensitivity is the fear of knowing what to say when a patient asks an awkward existential question, such as 'Why me?' or 'What have I done to deserve this?' This type of searching can challenge the nurse, bringing into question his or her own personal spirituality or philosophies surrounding life, death and religion. It would appear that spiritual care extends nursing beyond task focus and demands nurses to give of themselves and develop relationships, not just to perform tasks.

Emotionally demanding and fear-provoking

The information presented in relation to the intrinsic barriers indicates that there is an emotional cost or labour involved in the provision of spiritual care in that it can be emotionally and spiritually demanding. The material presented throughout this book indicates that many aspects associated with spirituality are deeply personal; indeed some issues are emotionally charged such as those pertaining to religion or matters concerning the sanctity of life. These areas can be extremely difficult for nurses to address since they can arouse our own personal fears that shape our attitudes and opinions. The fear of mismanagement or making a wrong judgement in difficult situations can lead to avoidance or denial that a patient has a particular spiritual need(s) that requires attention. Case study 5.2 shows how the nurse may have to play an arbitrary role – acting as advocate for the spiritual needs of the patient as well as being sensitive to the spiritual needs of immediate family and friends. Salladay & McDonnell (1989 p. 543) write:

A skilled patient advocate is a nurse who is first able and willing to set aside personal agendas and unit politics to participate with patients in their search for meaning during times that patients may be suffering, vulnerable, or frustrated.

This quotation implies that the role of advocate is fundamental when supporting patients in their decision making. Read Case study 5.2, paying particular attention to those factors that may place an emotional burden upon the nurse or health care team.

Having read the case study you have probably identified correctly that there are many ethical issues operating in this situation. With respect to Mr Francis' spiritual needs, he has come to a conscious decision that life is no longer worth living. There is a need to be aware that depression is a major compli-

Case study 5.2   In whose interest?

Mr Francis was admitted to the ward having suffered a very dense left-sided CVA (cerebrovascular accident, or stroke). For two days he was deeply unconscious and unresponsive, and was given intravenous fluids for hydration. Several days passed and slowly Mr Francis gained consciousness and became more alert. Prior to admission he had been a very active man who had had an excellent quality of life, free of any major illness or hospitalization. Mr Francis' wife and family stayed with him and supported him throughout the acute phase of the illness. Mr Francis' condition improved, and the process of rehabilitation was initiated. It soon became apparent that Mr Francis was aphasic, having a marked dysphagia. It was decided by the medical and nursing staff, in consultation with Mr Francis and his family, to pass a fine bore nasogastric tube and to commence enteral feeding. However, Mr Francis showed dissatisfaction with this by pulling out the tube. Again the tube was passed, and again Mr Francis pulled out the tube, to the displeasure of his family.

The nurses and consultant caring for Mr Francis discussed the matter with him, and it emerged that he did not want to be fed. However, when his family were present he would change his mind in an attempt to keep the peace. Mr Francis' family was rightly concerned that he would possibly starve to death, and asked for a gastrostomy tube to be inserted. Mr Francis agreed and consented to have the procedure performed. Several days later he pulled out the gastrostomy tube, and categorically refused to have it reinserted. Again when approached by the consultant and nursing staff Mr Francis indicated non-verbally that he did not want the gastrostomy tube reinserting. The consultant explained, in detail, informing him of the consequences of his decision, and that he would die if he were left without nutritional support. Mr Francis was adamant in his decision, and even persuasion from his family failed. Consequently Mr Francis died some days later.

cation affecting individuals who have suffered a stroke. Depression had been assessed for and excluded in Mr Francis' situation. However, he is faced with a dilemma – 'torn between the devil and the deep blue sea'. He is possibly thinking that his quality of life will never be the same. Yet Mr Francis is conscious of the needs of his family and the impact that his decision will have upon them. The case study indicates that Mr Francis's family is faced with the potential death of a loved one. It would appear that Mr Francis has made a conscious decision to die by not wanting to be enterally fed. However, he seeks to keep the peace and placate his family by following their wishes and instructions when they are present. In such situations the nurse may experience divided loyalties – wanting to act as advocate for the patient at the same time appreciating the helplessness, grief and spiritual

Activity 5.2 My personal space

Mr Singh Bhuller is a practising Sikh. The wearing of religious symbols and prayer are fundamental. Mr Singh is concerned that his customs and daily rituals will not be maintained while in hospital.

You are the admitting nurse working on a busy, general surgical ward. Can you identify any extrinsic barriers that may prevent Mr Singh from observing his religious practices while in your care?

distress that loved ones may be feeling when faced with such dilemmas.

These situations can place an emotional and spiritual strain upon all those involved. The nurse may need to act as an arbitrator, advocate between the patient and their family. Disagreement may occur between healthcare workers as to the appropriateness of the course of action chosen. The final outcome should be determined and made by the patient themselves since it is their spiritual needs that are paramount overriding the needs of others involved in the situation.

The antagonism and division one can experience in such situations can deplete one's own emotional and spiritual reserve – causing anxiety and fear. The ever-growing threat of complaint and litigation can further compound such situations. Questions like 'Did we take the appropriate course of action?' or 'Did we act in the best interests of individuals?' may be asked, especially when situations are complex involving and affecting the perceptions and opinions of several individuals.

EXTRINSIC FACTORS

This section will focus upon the category of barriers termed extrinsic – you may recall that these barriers are those external to an individual. Read Activity 5.2 and answer the question that follows.

You may have identified several extrinsic or environmental barriers that may prevent Mr Singh from maintaining his religious customs and practices, making sense of his illness and hospitalization:

lack of personal space
environmental distractions/interruptions

> **Box 5.3**   Extrinsic barriers
>
> **Organizational and management**
> **Environmental distractions resulting in loss of privacy**
> **Economic constraints**
>   Shortages of staff
>   Lack of time
> **Educational issues**
> **Reduced length of stay in hospital**
> **Not directly relevant to area of practice**
> **Prevailing opinion within society**

prayer heard by other patients/staff on the ward
staff too busy to facilitate
perhaps religious needs not adequately assessed upon admission
uncertainty concerning religious needs of Mr Singh.

Some of these barriers are associated with lack of privacy. Others are determined by management or organizational structures such as insufficient staff, the way that patient care is organized, the resources available to address Mr Singh's spiritual needs, or lack of time due to the busy nature of the ward. All these barriers will determine the amount of time the nurses will be able to devote to Mr Singh's general and spiritual care. Box 5.3 presents a list of extrinsic barriers that have been identified by nurse researchers (Ross 1994, McSherry 1998). Compare this against your own list, noting any similarities or differences.

More emphasis is now being placed on the need for health care establishments providing care within diverse client groups to address and support the spiritual needs of all individuals – both consumers and providers. This reversal in trends has seen spirituality being placed on management's operations agenda within many National Health Service structures.

Organizational and management

If nurses are to provide effective spiritual care, then there is a need for management to address many of the extrinsic barriers identified. The growing evidence addressing the spiritual dimension needs to be reviewed and a model of best practice devised, implemented and evaluated at local and national levels. Management needs to accept some responsibility for the provision of spiritual care. This has been made explicit in the nine National Charter Standards (HMSO 1992). The importance of providing an environment and climate in which a patient's spiritual or religious beliefs are addressed should be the norm rather than a government expectation. Therefore nurses should alert management to any environmental, economic or educational barriers that prevent them from implementing or addressing patients' spiritual needs satisfactorily, thus influencing the overall standard of care provided. However, caution needs to be exercised because managerial and organizational constraints could be used as an excuse for not getting involved.

Environmental distractions resulting in loss of privacy

Environmental barriers are ultimately determined by the context in which all care is to be provided. In the past acute sector care was provided on large 'Nightingale wards' where it was hard to maintain privacy or personal space. Privacy in such situations is gained by pulling round a curtain screen. This screen does preserve dignity but does not prevent personal conversations from being overheard. In such situations patients may not divulge personal information for fear that neighbouring patients are listening. It is hard to maintain confidentiality under such circumstances. Such problems may be overcome if the number of quiet rooms where patients could be counselled privately were increased.

It could be argued that many modern hospitals are much better suited to the needs of patients in respect of preserving dignity and affording privacy. Many areas now within the acute and private sectors have single rooms in which patients can be counselled or admitted in private, keeping distractions and interruptions to a minimum.

Economic constraints

Possibly the greatest obstacle in the provision of spiritual care, within the acute sectors, is lack of time and the restricted availability of staff (McSherry 1997). The contemporary health care system has changed drastically, witnessing an increase in

Caution

The lack of time could be seen as an excuse for not becoming involved. Spiritual care can be provided within the context of general care. The interactions that take place when bathing a patient or dressing a wound can be used to build trust and offer spiritual support.

patient expectation alongside a dramatic reduction in numbers of doctors and nurses. The result has seen medical and nursing staff providing care in situations that are highly stressful and demanding. In such situations spiritual care is seen as a low priority when contrasted against other more life-saving situations. The qualified nurse cannot be expected to provide spiritual care if he or she does not have the time to communicate or listen effectively.

It could be argued that the government has responded to this urgent need with recent pay incentives and the publication of the document *Making a difference: strengthening the nursing, midwifery and health visiting contribution to health and health care* (Department of Health 1999). However, it could be argued that this is not a long-term solution but rather a short-term remedy to try and reverse the worrying trend that afflicts the delivery of health care in many hospitals. The accumulative effect of recent trends, for example shortage of nurses and junior doctors and over-reliance upon bank staff, must bring into question the overall quality of care being provided. Therefore when qualified nurses report that they are too busy to provide spiritual care this probably reflects the reality of the situation in which they work.

Cynics may offer a counter-argument by stating that spiritual care is not something different from the 'general care' provided by nurses. Therefore the claims that we are 'too busy' or 'do not have sufficient time or staff' are redundant. Management are aware that to deliver a high standard of care requires commitment from staff who are highly trained and skilled within their chosen specialty. The same principle must be applied to the provision of spiritual care. The spiritual needs of patients will not be adequately addressed if they are left to chance.

Educational issues

Educational debates surrounding the spiritual dimension are addressed in more detail in Chapter 7. However, one major barrier that has been identified by numerous research studies is that nurses feel inadequately prepared to meet the spiritual needs of their patients (Boutell & Bozett 1990, Waugh 1992, Narayanasamy 1993). McSherry's (1997) survey revealed that some nurses did not feel confident in addressing a patient's spiritual needs because of a lack of insight or knowledge of this aspect of care.

Reduced length of stay in hospital

Within the acute sector the average stay in hospital is around 48 hours. This has been greatly reduced by advances in surgical procedures, screening, and new investigative techniques. These advances have to be viewed positively since they reduce the stress placed on individuals as a result of extensive hospitalization. However, this reduction in the length of stay may mean patients' spiritual needs are left unmet. Rapid turnover or throughput of patients means the opportunity may not exist for nurses to establish a trusting relationship in which a patient may reveal a spiritual need. Likewise nurses may be too concerned or preoccupied with outcome measures and bed occupancy figures, resulting in spiritual care being afforded low priority. Turner (1996 p. 60) recognizes that this dilemma may also be affecting hospice care:

Even in hospice care the process of bureaucratisation has produced a growing preoccupation with throughput, outcomes and cost-effectiveness, hence a concern for doing with little or no emphasis on being.

These concerns may not always affect care that is provided within the community or primary care settings, where practitioners have the opportunity and time to establish relationships that may extend over a period of weeks, and in the case of some chronic illnesses, months or years. Likewise nurses working with individuals with learning disabilities may have the opportunity to establish a meaningful relationship with their clients or users of a service over an extended period of time. The opportunity to develop such relationships can prove very rewarding for the client and the nurse since both can learn and grow spiritually together (Males & Boswell 1990, Balkizas & O' Hare 1994).

Not directly relevant to area of practice

The relevance of nursing staff intervening and addressing patients' spiritual needs has been identified as a potential barrier (McCavery 1985, McSherry 1997). Nurses working within certain specialties such as intensive care units may find it difficult to provide spiritual care to individuals who are unconscious and being ventilated. Likewise nurses working within rehabilitation units may find it difficult to provide spiritual care to individuals in a persistent vegetative state. The barriers originate from the inability to communicate effectively in that communication may be one-sided and perceived as ineffective. Read Case study 5.3 and reflect upon how you might feel if you were the nurse caring for John.

It is easy to assume that individuals who are unconscious or unresponsive do not require spiritual care. This assumption usually stems from our inability to interact with the patient in a meaningful manner. Even the most experienced of nurses find it difficult to communicate with ease in such circumstances. However, these circumstances should not prevent nurses from providing patient-centred and holistic care, accepting that behind the seemingly motionless exterior lies a human being in whom resides a spirit that requires nurturing and caring.

Some nurses question the relevance and appropriateness of tinkering in this aspect of individuals' lives, suggesting that spiritual issues should be addressed or dealt with by the hospital chaplain. However, this is a grave misconception since

---

Case study 5.3

John, a 21-year-old mechanic, was knocked off his motor bike and sustained severe head injuries. Surgery was performed to remove a large subdural haematoma. John never regained consciousness and was diagnosed as being in a persistent vegetative state. After several months in the neurosurgical ward John was transferred to a rehabilitation unit for intensive stimulation and rehabilitation. Prior to his accident John used to enjoy socializing with his colleagues and friends. He was a keen musician, playing guitar in a local rock band.

it assumes that spirituality is solely concerned with the religious. This approach towards spirituality could be seen as a defence mechanism that prevents nurses from being involved in an aspect of care that can be challenging and threatening. The literature indicates that nurses are in a prime position to attend to the spiritual needs of their patients because of their 24-hour responsibilities. Merely to state that the spiritual dimension is not our responsibility can be construed as 'passing the buck'.

Prevailing opinions within society

Allen (1991 p. 52) implies that forces operating within society, or indeed within the nursing profession, may be a major - obstacle in the provision of spiritual care. Individual nurses may not want to be seen as nonconforming – going against popular opinion and belief. Involvement in an individual's spiritual care may result in other nurses making value judgements about a colleague's motives. Some may see a nurse who attends to the spiritual needs of patients as a fanatic – a 'Bible basher' – when in reality all the nurse is trying to do is provide total patient care. In such instances the nurse may provide spiritual care in secrecy or, sadly, the nurse may stop attending to the spiritual needs of patients because of fear of reprisal or recrimination. These anxieties are highlighted by Aveyard (1995 p. 44) when discussing the concept of self-disclosure within teaching:

But on the rare occasions when I have referred to instances relating to my faith, I sense that some students feel that it is inappropriate.

Therefore social desirability may be a force that inhibits the provision of spiritual care. Yet ideally we should see all qualified nurses, regardless of race, creed, colour or religion, attending to the spiritual needs of patients. In an ideal world this would mean we do not make value judgements about other individuals but use tolerance and common sense. There needs to be a sense of proportion. Likewise we would not want individuals with strong religious beliefs trying to convert or preaching to vulnerable patients.

Activity 5.3

Read this chapter again thinking specifically about any strategies or measures you could use to try and address some of these barriers within yourself or your ward environment.

No easy solutions

As indicated, it is all too easy to become prescriptive, stating that nurses should be providing spiritual care without giving due thought and attention to the demands and pressures that many nurses encounter in the course of their practice. However, it is all too easy to declare that we cannot do anything to remove these political and economic barriers until the wastage, attrition and recruitment problems that shroud the nursing profession are resolved. If we adopt this approach then many patients' spiritual needs in our care will be left unmet. Box 5.4 presents some steps that we may take to overcome some of the barriers that prevent nurses from providing spiritual care.

There is a need for us to inform management of shortfalls in staff levels that impinge on all aspects of care. We need to develop insight into our own spirituality and spiritual needs. By becoming spiritually aware we will be in a stronger position

---

Box 5.4 Steps we can take to remove the barriers

Intrinsic
    Self-awareness. Become more introspective, reflecting upon our own beliefs and attitudes, values. Think about our own spirituality. Question our attitudes to different groups, situations.
    Tolerance and patience. Respect those with different cultural, ethnic or religious principles instead of making value judgements.

Extrinsic
    Inform. Make management aware of any obstacles that inhibit us from delivering the quality of care that we strive to provide. This may be the lack of a quiet room on the ward or unit in which to talk privately with patients, or drawing attention to poor staffing levels and skills mix.
    Resources. Be aware of who the hospital chaplain(s) are and the service that they provide. We need to be aware of the resources at our disposal that can assist us in providing spiritual care such as information leaflets or books that offer insight into the customs and practices of different religions. Know where to contact an interpreter if required.

to recognize similar needs within our patients and colleagues. We need to be aware of our own personal fears and prejudices that may influence our attitudes to this dimension of care. By exploring our own personal beliefs and values we may better be able to tolerate and accept that we are all unique with diverse belief and value systems. Schoenbeck (1994) suggests that the key to effective spiritual care is respectfulness of the patient's belief system.

CONCLUSION

This chapter has introduced you to the numerous barriers, intrinsic and extrinsic, that may prevent nurses from delivering spiritual care. It has been stressed that there are many variables that must be considered before we accuse the nursing profession of failing to provide spiritual care. If the nursing profession adopts a judgemental and prescriptive attitude towards the delivery of spiritual care then it could be accused of double standards. This would be so because it would be failing to acknowledge the many pressures, political and economic, that may prevent nurses from attending to patients' spiritual needs. However, it is suggested that there are many measures we as nurses can adopt in order to remove some of the barriers that prevent us from providing spiritual care. By far the greatest measure we can take is to develop our own spiritual awareness, which will enable us to remove many of the intrinsic barriers. Once we have put our own house in order, then we can turn our attention to the extrinsic barriers that exist within practice.

REFERENCES

Allen C 1991 The inner light. Nursing Standard 5 (20): 52–53
Aveyard B 1995 A question of faith. Nursing Standard 9 (5): 44
Balkizas D, O'Hare M 1994 The healing hand of God. Nursing Standard 9 (9): 46–47
Boutell K A, Bozett F W 1990 Nurses' assessment of patients' spirituality: continuing education implications. Journal of Continuing Education in Nursing 21 (4): 172–176
Clark C C, Cross J R, Deane D M, Lowry L W 1991 Spirituality: integral to quality care. Holistic Nursing Practice 5 (3): 67–76

Department of Health 1999 Making a difference: strengthening the nursing, midwifery and health visiting contribution to health and health care. HMSO, London

Harrison J 1993 Spirituality and nursing practice. Journal of Clinical Nursing 2: 211–217

HMSO 1992 The patient's charter. HMSO, London

Males J, Boswell C 1990 Spiritual needs of people with a mental handicap. Nursing Standard 4 (48): 35–37

McCavery R 1985 Spiritual care in acute illness. In: McGilloway O, Myco F (eds) Nursing and spiritual care. Harper & Row, London

McSherry W 1996 Raising the spirits. Nursing Times 92 (3): 48–49

McSherry W 1997 A descriptive survey of nurses' perceptions of spirituality and spiritual care. Unpublished MPhil thesis, University of Hull, Hull

McSherry W 1998 Nurses' perceptions of spirituality and spiritual care. Nursing Standard 13 (4): 36–40

Narayanasamy A 1993 Nurses' awareness and educational preparation in meeting their patients' spiritual needs. Nurse Education Today 13 (3): 196–201

Ross L 1994 Spiritual care: the nurse's role. Nursing Standard 8 (33): 33–37

Ross L 1997 The nurse's role in assessing and responding to patients' spiritual needs. International Journal of Palliative Nursing 3 (1): 37–42

Salladay S A, McDonnell M M 1989 Spiritual care, ethical choices and patient advocacy. Nursing Clinics of North America 24 (2): 543–549

Schoenbeck S L 1994 Called to care: addressing the spiritual needs of patients. Journal of Practical Nursing 44 (3): 19–23

Soeken K L, Carson V B 1987 Responding to the spiritual needs of the chronically ill. Nursing Clinics of North America 22 (3): 603–611

Sommer D R 1989 The spiritual needs of dying children. Issues in Comprehensive Paediatric Nursing 12 (2/3): 225–230

Taylor J E, Highfield M, Amenta M 1994 Attitudes and beliefs regarding spiritual care. Cancer Nursing 17 (6): 479–487

Turner P 1996 Caring more, doing less. Nursing Times 92 (34): 59–60

Waugh L A 1992 Spiritual aspects of nursing: a descriptive study of nurses' perceptions. Unpublished PhD thesis, Queen Margaret College, Edinburgh

FURTHER READING

These articles will further develop your understanding of the barriers, intrinsic and extrinsic, that may affect nurses' ability to provide spiritual care. These articles are informative and interesting to read. By reflecting upon their content you will gain a deeper insight into many of the issues addressed in the chapter.

Allen C 1991 The inner light. Nursing Standard 5 (20): 52–53

Aveyard B 1995 A question of faith. Nursing Standard 9 (5): 44

Harrison J 1993 Spirituality and nursing practice. Journal of Clinical Nursing 2: 211–217

Ross L 1994 Spiritual care: the nurse's role. Nursing Standard 8 (33): 33–37

Turner P 1996 Caring more, doing less. Nursing Times 92 (34): 59–60

6

Skills required to provide spiritual care

INTRODUCTION

This chapter will review the different skills nurses require in order to assess, plan, implement and evaluate spiritual care. At this stage in the book you are probably recognizing that the concept of spirituality is subjective, diverse and unique to each individual. The subjective nature of the spiritual dimension means that nurses require a broad range of skills for them to overcome many of the barriers that can prevent the provision of spiritual care. By utilizing these skills and developing their own self-awareness nurses will be in a stronger position to act as

Food for thought

This, then is the challenge in nursing the spiritually distressed person: to listen, to accept, to explore and finally, to offer no ready answers. This is clearly a difficult task but a rewarding one. In the end, persons who discover their own meaning and their own reason for believing in what they do will usually be the more satisfied. The nurse's task is not to get in the way of that process taking place. But equally and almost paradoxically, it is the nurse's task to become involved with the dispirited person. The balance between standing back and becoming immersed is a difficult one to achieve. It is also, a very human and important one. (Burnard 1987 p. 381) advocates for their patients who present with spiritual need(s). The chapter demonstrates the need for multidisciplinary collaboration in the provision of spiritual care. It is argued that no single professional body has a monopoly with respect to the spiritual dimension.

The quotation from Burnard highlights the subtle nature of spiritual care. It reveals that spiritual care is not easy, and at times is uncomfortable, indeed a challenge. The quotation implies that there are right and wrong methods to be utilized in this aspect of care. Fundamentally the quotation indicates that the area of spiritual care is a two-way process that can enrich the lives of both the patient and the nurse. However, if spiritual care is to be effective and the dispirited person and the nurse are to benefit from the interactions, then there are certain skills or guiding principles to be followed.

IDENTIFYING THE SKILLS

In order to proceed with this chapter there is a need to identify the skills that may be required by nurses to support and facilitate spiritual care. Read the following case study and spend several minutes reflecting upon the skills you would require in order to meet the patient's spiritual needs.

You may have identified several skills that are necessary to support Vincent and to meet his spiritual needs. You will have recognized the need for good interpersonal skills in helping you to address Vincent's immediate concerns. The questions that Vincent expresses are existential; questioning his reason

---

Case study 6.1   Questioning meaning and purpose

Vincent is 38 years of age and works as a business executive with an international company. He has been married for 10 years and has three young children, all under six. He is a little overweight and smokes around 10 cigarettes per day. His wife has been encouraging Vincent to slow down but with little success. Life operates around Vincent's need to meet deadlines and production targets. Early one morning he is woken by a tightness around his chest and a pain radiating down his left arm and up into his jaw. His wife phones for an ambulance and Vincent is rushed into hospital diagnosed as a myocardial infarction. You are the nurse responsible for Vincent's care. The day after admission in conversation he says to you, 'My life will never be the same' and 'What will I do about work and who will support my family?'

for living, indicating that you may require some insight into what constitutes spirituality. A comprehensive list of skills required to enable Vincent to achieve total well-being are listed in Box 6.1. It must be stressed that these skills are not used in isolation. The biggest danger of identifying lists is that we assume each skill is separate from the next, not connected or used in conjunction with the others. If you observe skilled practitioners you will see that they draw upon their knowledge and use all their skills in an integrated manner. The skills and knowledge become an integral part of the person. These skills are drawn upon to resolve an issue or concern. The same principle applies when supporting individuals with spiritual needs. The provision of spiritual care must become a natural part of the practitioner's experience or else the care will be fragmented and unnatural – rather like using a checklist when a vehicle has been booked in for an MOT test. McCavery (1985 p. 139) alerts us to this fact:

However, spiritual activity can never be restricted to mere religious practice, nor can spiritual needs be fulfilled successfully in a scientific, planned way.

Perhaps while examining the skills listed you may feel that many nurses already possess such skills, which are developed to a high standard and used frequently in their clinical practice.

To assume that all nurses are not able to deal with patient's spiritual needs is presumptuous and judgemental. One cannot generalize and say that nurses are not able to meet their patients' spiritual needs. Such a generalization would be misleading, contradicting current research findings (Waugh 1992, Harrison 1993, Narayanasamy 1993, McSherry 1997). An excerpt from McSherry's thesis (1997 p. 127) supports this

---

Box 6.1 Skills required to provide spiritual care

Good interpersonal and communication skills
Development of trust
Sensitivity
Self-awareness – clarification of personal values
Provision of support to the patient and colleagues
Education and training
Openness and honesty
Multidisciplinary collaboration
Recognition of your own limitations

> **Caution**
>
> Caution must be exercised when identifying and discussing the types of skills that nurses may require to meet spiritual needs. The danger is to assume that nurses do not already possess them. When teaching nurses about spiritual care, I conclude my session by stating: 'Nurses already possess many skills required to take the initiative in dealing with patients' spiritual needs. What they sometimes lack is the confidence and education.'

point, indicating that nurses are recognizing patients presenting with a spiritual need(s):

Of the nurses surveyed 465 (84.7%) stated that they had encountered a patient(s) with a spiritual need(s). A limitation of this question is that there is no means of identifying how frequently, or how recently the nurse had identified such a need(s). Of the qualified nurses surveyed 219 (39.9%) felt that they were able to meet their patient's spiritual needs. A limitation in relation to this question is that specific needs were not asked for or identified.

However, there is no room for complacency because only a small percentage of qualified nurses felt they were able to meet their patients' spiritual need(s) successfully. In several research studies (Waugh 1992, Narayanasamy 1993, McSherry 1997) nurses have asked for more education regarding addressing the spiritual dimension of care. This recognition of their own limitations indicates that nurses feel a little uncertain about how to address this aspect of care. This uncertainty may arise because they feel that they do not have sufficient insight or skills to address the spiritual dimension.

COMMUNICATION/INTERPERSONAL SKILLS

It could be argued that communication and interpersonal skills are fundamental to all aspects of nursing. Without the use of good interpersonal skills and communication important information may not be conveyed between patient and nurse or nurse and other professionals. Given the deeply sensitive and personal nature of spirituality, there is a greater need for communication to be effective in removing barriers and alleviating

---

Box 6.2 Terms defined

Attentive listening
  This means listening to and not necessarily saying anything as the patient discloses his or her spiritual need. It is about paying attention to words, tone of voice and non-verbal language. Attentive listening is not a shallow activity but one that allows you to engage with the patient at a deeper level.
Non-verbal communication
  The area of non-verbal communication is crucial in generating a therapeutic relationship between nurse and patient. Nurses must have an insight into the non-verbal gestures, expressions and body language that they display. They must be able to observe the non-verbal cues exhibited by patients.
Presence, or making time
  By far the greatest consolation an individual can have when experiencing a spiritual concern is knowing that someone is there for him or her in this time of need. Presence means being with the individual in a physical and psychological sense.

---

fears. It would appear that effective communication is a prerequisite to the formation of any kind of relationship (McCavery 1985). Without the use of good communication we can never expect to know, understand, or become aware of individuals' innermost fears, motives or spiritual concerns.

When addressing an individual's spiritual needs the nurse must use all forms of communication and interpersonal skills to identify and evaluate the problem. It is not the intention of this section to explore all aspects of communication, but rather to identify methods that are important when attending to patients' spiritual concerns. Three important aspects of communication that seem pertinent to the issue of spiritual care are attentive listening, non-verbal communication, and the use of presence (Box 6.2).

Attentive listening

A brief definition of attentive listening is provided. However, there is more to attentive listening than merely paying attention. We can give all the indications to a patient that we are listening when in reality we hear little about what they have expressed. Burnard (1988 p. 371) warns us of this hidden danger:

The first practical step in helping others with spiritual problems, then, is listening to them. This may seem so obvious as to not need stating. However we often spend considerable time with others rehearsing our replies to what they are saying, rather than truly listening to them.

It would appear that attentive listening is about focusing upon what the patient has to say, clearing our head of any judgements, ideas or opinions that we have concerning the problem, thereby giving our undivided attention. In situations that are intense and stressful there is a tendency for us to fill the silence. However, silence can be a powerful tool in that it allows individuals to think, reflect and process points that may have been raised. When facilitating workshops on spiritual care it is always tempting to fill natural silences with speech, especially if the content of what was being discussed prior to the silence was emotionally challenging. Morrison (1992) tells us that possibly the best form of communication is silence.

Narayanasamy (1997) provides a list of attributes of a good listener. These are summarized here:

Generating an environment and counselling relationship in which the patient feels he or she is being listened to.

Giving your complete attention to the patient. Suspending your own thoughts and opinions on the subject – clearing your own head.

Using reflection and paraphrasing to indicate you are giving full attention, and listening hard.

Responding warmly to the patient. Using open gestures and speech to encourage the patient to talk, indicating acceptance of his or her spiritual need.

It must be stressed that attentive listening is difficult. This particular skill is not developed overnight but through much experience and practice. The use of prolonged attentive listening can be demanding, resulting in the nurse feeling exhausted. This is because such interventions require the nurse to enter into a relationship that draws upon his or her own spiritual reserves. Therefore attentive listening is not easy because it is time-consuming and demanding. However, the benefits of simply listening to and allowing patients to express their inner concerns, fears and spiritual needs can in itself be therapeutic. As part of listening the nurse may also be observing for other non-verbal cues that indicate the patient has a spiritual need.

Activity 6.1

Consider the points that have been raised in this section regarding attentive listening. Write down what attributes are to be found in a good listener. Can you think of any ways in which we can improve our listening skills?

Non-verbal communication

The importance of observation was stressed in the section addressing assessment (Chapter 4). An important part of assessment is being alert to factors or cues that may be suggestive of a patient having spiritual need(s). McSherry (1996) recalls how a patient's non-verbal behaviours indicated a deep spiritual need.

Case study 6.2

A patient was withdrawn, used limited communication and detached herself from any form of interaction with other patients. It emerged after several days that the patient had experienced a great loss and needed time to grieve and reconcile, adjusting to the loss. This resulted in her displaying the non-verbal cues that the nurses interpreted as odd. The nurses reacted to the cues in a judgemental manner, viewing the patient's behaviour as antagonistic. The patient was immediately labelled unpopular (Stockwell 1984).

This brief case study illustrates the importance of nurses being alert to the unspoken words of patients. It warns us of the danger of attaching the wrong interpretation to different non-verbal behaviours displayed by individuals. If we observe a patient adopting the fetal position because of a severe abdominal pain we would not dismiss this and say 'it is trapped wind' and provide no analgesia to assist in alleviating the pain and discomfort. A fundamental principle in pain management is you always believe the pain is what the patient tells you. A major principle we need to remember in the management of spiritual pain is never to make value judgements based on our interpretations of non-verbal behaviours. Elsdon (1995 p. 642) illustrates this when addressing the concept of spiritual pain:

The cure for physical pain may be analgesia, but the cure for spiritual pain is to be found in the experience of the pain itself. Spiritual pain, then, is not so much a 'problem to be solved,' as a 'question to be lived', and thus demands different qualities in health-care professionals.

We have indicated that communication is a two-way process – an interaction between for example the nurse and the patient. There is a need for nurses and all health care professionals involved in the provision of spiritual care to be aware of their own non-verbal language. The amount of appropriate eye contact given during an interaction when dealing with a patient presenting with a spiritual need can convey the professional's level of concern and empathy. For example a consultant who walks into the consulting room to break bad news and is constantly looking at the clock on the wall does not convey empathy or sensitivity to the individual's needs. Likewise the junior doctor who informs relatives that a loved one has died while standing with his or her arms folded and backed up against the wall does not inspire confidence.

When providing spiritual care a conscious awareness of our non-verbal signals is required. The way in which the nurse sits can encourage the patient to feel at ease and relaxed. Adopting an open posture (arms and legs not crossed) and sitting in a relaxed manner, leaning slightly towards the individual, will encourage dialogue (Burnard 1988). It must be stressed that such skills do not develop overnight, and neither do they develop through a process of osmosis in the classroom environment, although this can be a useful training ground. Counselling skills only become a natural and spontaneous part of the nurse after considerable use in practice. It is worth remembering that we are all beginners and mistakes will be made (Morrison 1992). However, it is how we reflect and learn from our experiences that is important and developmental.

Developing trust

Patients will not disclose their spiritual needs in an environment that is alien, unfriendly or hostile. In fact effective spiritual care can only be provided in an environment that is totally the opposite. Patients need to feel that nurses can be trusted with their spiritual needs. Trust will only be established

> **Box 6.3**   A simple illustration
>
> A patient asks you for a jug of water. You are busy because of staff shortages. Your immediate response to the patient is 'I will be back in a minute'. The nurse's minute must be the longest minute on earth. Perhaps several hours later you remember the patient's request, but by then it is too late and someone else has satisfied his or her thirst. My response to such a request is to fetch the water immediately, if I am not undertaking a task of greater priority. The patient is satisfied and forms an impression of you based on reliability and dependability. If patients feel that they can trust you in simple matters, like filling a jug of water, then they will trust you in matters of greater importance.

if patients feel that a nurse is both reliable and dependable. When undertaking workshops on spirituality, a question I am frequently asked is 'Why do patients disclose their spiritual needs to you?' After spending many years pondering upon this question, my response is 'Patients feel that they can trust me and that I am dependable and reliable'. Further reflection into why a patient may perceive these qualities in me is because I try to make time for them in meeting simple everyday requests (Box 6.3). The illustration may be verging on the ridiculous, but this approach is what I feel encourages patients to disclose personal and sensitive needs to me. Narayanasamy (1997 p. 215) confirms this, writing:

Trust grows over a period of time as the client tests the environment, risks self-disclosure, and observes the carer's adherence to commitment.

Patients are not passive recipients of care; they are constantly assessing the situation and undertaking a personal audit of the skills and services available in a particular area. They assess the qualities that individual members of staff display (obviously this process is not undertaken if the patient is unconscious or has a cognitive impairment), reaching an opinion based on their own judgements and expectations. This is a possible reason why certain nurses are used frequently by patients to disclose their innermost concerns. Trust-building is a skill that can be developed by all nurses. It only takes a minute to sow the seeds of trust and respect. Trust can be developed by utilizing the other skills addressed in previous sections.

Sensitivity

Spiritual care cannot be provided if the nurse is not sensitive to the needs of individual patients. Spirituality has been explored within the context of holism (Chapter 3). This discussion demonstrated that we are all unique individuals made up of many interactive systems, which are constantly changing and developing according to environmental, political, social and economic forces. Therefore, individuals and their spirituality are constantly changing and evolving – adapting to different circumstances, both positive and negative, across the lifespan. Therefore it is highly unlikely that a nurse will encounter two patients with exactly the same spiritual need.

A nurse may have to address spiritual needs stemming from deep-rooted conflict, unresolved anger, frustration or guilt. All of these may have affected the individual's system for months or years. Such spiritual needs must be handled in a sensitive manner without judgement being passed (Case study 4.6). Likewise the nurse may have to support patients who have been diagnosed with a terminal disease, helping them prepare for death (Schoenbeck 1994, Elsdon 1995).

For some individuals their spirituality may be shaped and expressed through formal religious affiliation and worship. Nurses may have to assist individuals in maintaining their religious practices while in hospital. Religion is a very sensitive subject that can arouse strong emotions. Some individuals, both nurse and patient, can become very protective of their own personal beliefs if they feel these are being challenged or brought into question. Therefore matters of religion must be dealt with sensitively by nurses and other health care professionals. Perhaps what makes matters of religion difficult to

---

Case study 6.3 A need for sensitivity

Victoria is admitted to your ward with a suspected drug overdose of heroin. She is a single parent, having three young children to three different fathers. Victoria earns money by working as a prostitute in the city. The medical team stabilizes Victoria's condition and after several days in hospital she makes a full recovery. In the mean time her children have been fostered out to other families by social services. Victoria is annoyed and frustrated at the interventions by social services and is concerned that her children will not be returned to her because this is her third suicide attempt within three months.

address is that they can challenge our own personal beliefs and values about the meaning of life and existence (Burnard 1988).

Read Case study 6.3 and write down any areas that you feel would require sensitive handling.

The case study contains several issues – addiction, prostitution, overdose, fostering of children – that if not dealt with sensitively could turn the situation into a confrontation. It is evident that Victoria is experiencing a great deal of turbulence in her life and is searching for support and meaning. The biggest danger is that some nurses may make a judgement based on her heroin addiction and her prostitution – viewing her as a loser. Such an evaluation would be unsafe and unfair because we are not aware of all the variables in the equation that may have resulted in Victoria taking the path into drugs and prostitution. The correct way of addressing this situation is to ensure that Victoria receives the same spiritual care as any other patient on the ward. We should be making no distinctions based on her lifestyle or history. The case study highlights that if nurses are to be successful in this challenge, then they need to be in touch with their own personal beliefs and values (Burnard 1988, Harrison 1993, Narayanasamy 1997).

Honesty

No communication will be effective if a relationship is not based upon honesty and trust. The area of spiritual care is no exception – it requires the nurse delivering spiritual care to be honest and open. If a patient finds that individuals have not been open and honest about aspects of care and diagnosis and the truth is eventually revealed, then the patient concerned can be left feeling hurt and alone, adding further to a dispirited state. McCavery (1985 p. 140) writes:

It is difficult to imagine any aspect of nursing where truth is more important than in the area of spiritual care. Yet half-truths, or even lies, are often commonplace in respect of patients with poor prognosis. Phrases such as 'Of course you're going to get better', or 'don't be worried, you'll be home in no time', come from professionals and relatives alike.

Read Case study 6.4 and write down how you might have handled this situation. Pay particular attention to possible reasons why professionals and family may find it difficult to tell the truth.

One reason why professionals may not want to tell the truth is fear of causing distress to the patient. By dressing up bad news in ambiguous language it protects the individual from the full force of reality. An example of this is saying 'You have a growth'. This also shields the professional, acting as a defence mechanism. These factors may be operating in Case study 6.4. Frank's family are trying to protect him from the reality of the situation by seeking alternative ways of addressing the question of his anticipated death. Certainly they do not want to cause him any distress, given his current condition. However, the chances are that Frank is very much aware of his situation. This form of deception can destroy trust, especially if an individual suspects that things are not what they seem and insists on answers. When the individual is made aware of the correct diagnosis he or she can feel angry and hurt, even betrayed. It is difficult for nurses because they are often arbitrators with limited power, having to respect the authority of the consultant while acting as advocate for the patient. However, this relationship is changing and nurses are often present when bad news is given and in some areas of work nurses actually take the lead in this area.

The old maxim 'honesty is the best policy' certainly applies when addressing spiritual needs. Looking at the case study, how might you address this situation? You could contact the

---

Case study 6.4   To tell or not to tell?

Frank, aged 65, is rushed to the ward following resuscitation in the outpatient department. On admission to your ward Frank is semiconscious and the medical staff feel death is imminent. Frank's next of kin are notified and asked to come into the ward. However, the medical staff's prediction is proved wrong and several days later Frank is still alive, floating in and out of consciousness. The medical staff believe that Frank's present condition is the result of an abdominal tumour. One afternoon while on duty you notice that Frank's relative is a little anxious and concerned. Upon enquiry the relative reveals that Frank is a practising Roman Catholic and the relative would like his priest to come and administer the sacrament of the sick. However, the relative is aware that Frank, despite his strong faith, is still fearful of death. The relative is also unsure about whether to tell Frank about his diagnosis and prognosis.

How might you address this situation?

Roman Catholic chaplain and ask him to do a general visit to the ward. This approach may not distress Frank, who may think that the priest visits the ward as a matter of course. Alternatively, you might consult Frank when conscious and ask him what he wants and what he feels. This latter approach would do more to promote trust and honesty – especially if Frank were to recover.

Self-awareness

Self-awareness is fundamental to the fostering of relationships that will prove effective in meeting patients' spiritual needs. Several authors (Burnard 1988, Harrison 1993, Narayanasamy 1997) underline the importance of developing personal awareness of one's own beliefs and values when providing spiritual care. McSherry (1996 p. 49) writes:

Spiritual awareness does not imply religiosity or piety, but the ability to explore positively one's own attitudes and feelings about matters that are fundamental to our existence.

The quotation indicates that there is a need for all nurses to have insight or self-awareness of their own beliefs and values. Self-awareness or personal value clarification is not just for the religious but is applicable to all health care professionals. Like many of the other skills mentioned in this chapter, self-awareness requires nurturing and developing. Our self-awareness can change as our values, beliefs or attitudes change through exposure to different situations or events that may occur in life or practice. Self-awareness can be developed through training. Self-awareness concerns the development and acknowledgement of our own inner thoughts, feelings and behaviours. This insight is important if we are to accept and understand ourselves. Without this personal understanding and insight we are probably less likely to be able to understand others (Burnard 1988, Narayanasamy 1997, Ross 1997). By fostering our own spiritual awareness we will be more focused and receptive to those who may have a spiritual concern (Schoenbeck 1994, Elsdon 1995). Ross (1997 p. 167) identified the association between self-awareness and the delivery of spiritual care:

Firstly, concerning the nurse, it seemed that nurses who demonstrated a personal search for meaning in their own lives, although they identified a narrow range of spiritual needs, gave spiritual care at a deeper level than those who did not demonstrate this characteristic.

Ross's conclusions reinforce the need for nurses to develop self-awareness or else the type of spiritual care provided may not go beyond superficial enquiry into religious affiliation (although necessary), which does not constitute spiritual care at a deeper level.

Three methods that can be used to generate self-awareness are reflection, critical analysis and appraisal of oneself and experiences (Fig. 6.1). Reflection is normally a retrospective activity – thinking about the event or incident after it has passed. Reflection is about reviewing a situation, questioning one's thoughts, feelings or personal actions. We can all reflect upon situations but we may not act upon what we have learned or discovered. Critical analysis is looking at a situation in more detail. It is not merely reflecting upon the situation but implies reviewing and considering all aspects in a balanced manner. Critical appraisal is more in-depth and structured than reflection. Appraisal is usually performed by a third party. We may ask a colleague to observe our actions or responses in a particular situation and provide verbal or written feedback. These three methods provide us with an insight into our behaviours, feelings and attitudes. If we use one in isolation from the rest we may only become aware of ourselves in monochrome. If we use two methods we may see more detail and the picture will be in colour. By employing all three methods we build up a

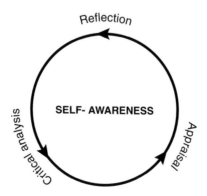

Figure 6.1 Methods that can develop self-awareness.

'3D' picture of ourselves, our emotions and our feelings and in this way become self-aware.

However, one fundamental ingredient is required in utilizing any of these methods – time alone. We can only truly find and understand ourselves by going into our own inner wilderness. We cannot find ourselves in the constant bustle of modern living. Solitude and stillness are necessary if the individual is to enter into a dialogue with self. This is evident in the writings of many religious or spiritual leaders who, in order to find themselves, physically withdrew from the world, isolating themselves from material distractions. Obviously this method is not being advocated. However, the principle of spending time alone for 5 minutes a day reflecting, critically analysing situations or questioning our actions to a particular patient or event will develop self-awareness.

There are other methods that can be helpful in developing self-awareness. Harrison & Burnard (1993) advocate the use of a 'Spiritual values clarification questionnaire', which can be completed by individuals undertaking workshops on spirituality. The questionnaire encourages the individual to focus upon self, questioning personal beliefs, values and attitudes towards spirituality. The questionnaire is a useful activity for encouraging debate and dialogue.

In summary, self-awareness is essential to our own spiritual and personal growth. It would be a grave error to assume that only the methods mentioned in this section can develop self-awareness. There are many different exercises that can lead to individuals developing self-awareness. Once aware of the need for self-awareness, many people use methods or exercises that suit their own personalities and social circumstances.

Activity 6.2 Having a go

Spend 5 minutes, alone, in a quiet place reflecting upon an event or incident that involved you. Ask yourself several questions – How did I feel at the time? How do I feel now? Why did I feel that way? Could I have reacted any differently? What would I change if the situation reoccurred? What have I learned about myself and others?

SUPPORT

By now you will have realized that the provision of spiritual care is not easy in that it can be emotionally and spiritually draining. It is important to recognize that we are not alone in the provision of spiritual care. There is a need for support from colleagues and other health care professionals with whom we work (Burnard 1988). Counselling can be very demanding and individuals may find that they do not have sufficient skills or resources to address a patient's particular need. Sometimes a nurse and patient may have grown too close so that judgements are clouded or obscured. In such situations the nurse and the patient may require support from colleagues to work through the situation.

Collaboration

It is correct to state that no single professional group has the monopoly in relation to the provision of spiritual care (Stoter 1995). Nurses are in a unique position in that the nature of their work and their duty rostering means that they have contact with patients 24 hours a day, 7 days a week, 52 weeks a year. Stoter (1995 p. 137) emphasizes the unique and central role that the nurse plays as the facilitator of spiritual care:

It is important to make the point here that the prime responsibility for giving continuous spiritual care inevitably lies with the nursing staff who are there all the time. They are likely to be the key people, if not always, for the in-depth care at least as facilitators of that process with the responsibility to ensure that spiritual care is given.

However, this still does not mean that nurses are solely responsible for providing spiritual care. In fact research suggests nurses feel that a multidisciplinary approach is required if patients' spiritual needs are to be met (Waugh 1992, Narayanasamy 1993, Keighley 1997, McSherry 1997).

McSherry's (1997) results confirm that nurses do not perceive themselves as the main providers of spiritual care. Of the 549 nurses surveyed, 76.7% (421) felt that spiritual care should be provided by a combination of people. This combination included nurses, chaplains, patient, family, friends and the patient's own religious leader. The overwhelming response to this question indicates that the provision of spiritual care must be flexible and collaborative in that there must be an exchange of information in relation to spiritual care among all parties concerned.

Stoter (1995) urges caution, indicating that at the end of the day it is the patient or his or her relatives who will choose the key person in the delivery of spiritual care. It therefore appears that spiritual care should be managed through teamwork. A team approach to the management of spiritual care will ensure that everyone is working towards the same goal and outcome. However, it would appear that the nurse has a central role to play not only in the identification of such needs, but also in the facilitation of spiritual care.

Religious needs

Through collaboration and liaising with chaplains, patients who have a spiritual need(s) that stems from their affiliation with a formal religion can access support. Through collaboration such patients will receive expert advice and support. There may be occasions when a patient asks the nurse about a matter of theology or religious doctrine that the nurse is unable to address. In such instances the nurse can enlist the services of the hospital chaplain or the patient's own spiritual/religious leader.

Nurses need to be aware that the chaplain has a specific pastoral function to play. Chaplains are there not only to support patients in their time of need, but also are a valuable source of support to other health care workers. Many chaplains within National Health Service trusts are now termed 'ecumenical', that is they provide support to all religious denominations and are only too willing to offer support (Leggieri 1986, Speck 1992, Elsdon 1995).

The non-believer

With respect to the provision of spiritual care, nurses need to protect patients from religious zealots and sects who seek to convert vulnerable people. Nurses need to be on their guard against organizations that may access health care institutions with a view to converting or preaching to individuals who have no means of escape. Many trusts do not allow organizations access unless they have sought the appropriate approval. However, some do slip the through the net and nurses must be vigilant.

Another area that must be considered under this section of religious needs is the spiritual needs of the non-believer. Nurses must also address the spiritual needs of the atheist and agnostic. Assuming that spiritual care is only relevant to those who have a strong religious faith is misguided. Atheists and agnostics may still raise existential questions and be in need of spiritual care (Burnard 1988a). It is on such occasions that the nurse must provide care that is appropriate. Arranging a visit from the hospital chaplain could be perceived as offensive (McSherry 1996). The nurse will need to support such patients without the involvement of any religious organization.

RECOGNITION OF OUR OWN LIMITATIONS

One of the gravest mistakes nurses can make in supporting individuals with spiritual needs is not to acknowledge their limitations. To continue in an interaction with a patient that is beyond one's level of expertise or control is dangerous and potentially damaging. If a nurse feels that a situation has entered a different or difficult phase that is beyond his or her level of expertise, then this should be recognized and discussed between both parties involved. It is unrealistic to imagine that we have answers or solutions to every spiritual need that will be encountered – given the unique and personal nature of spirituality.

The nurse must therefore acknowledge this and be prepared to say to patients:

I am sorry but I have not got any answers to this question.

or

I can see that you still require support in this matter. However, I feel that I cannot help you any further but I can refer you on to someone who has a little more knowledge in this area.

This public acceptance of one's own limitations in no way constitutes failure. Carson (1989) and Harrison (1993) feel that this public acknowledgement constitutes humility, which is an essential element for personal spiritual growth.

Some authors have argued that nurses may not possess the skills to adequately address patients who are experiencing spiritual needs. Burnard (1988) and Harrison (1993) feel that for the spiritually distressed patient basic counselling skills are not enough. While this appears to be a criticism of nurses' abilities, the point does warrant further explanation. Burnard and Harrison are not being critical but are making a valid observation in that although nurses do possess some basic counselling skills, these may not be sufficient to help individuals with deep-rooted problems. Such individuals may require the release of emotions that will require regular contact with a counsellor over an extended period of time. Therefore nurses need to assess the full situation before entering into a counselling relationship with patients who have spiritual needs. Conversely, Burnard and Harrison's observation does not act as an 'opt out' clause since they are alerting nurses to the hidden traps, not stating that nurses should not provide spiritual care.

CONCLUSION

This chapter has introduced you to some of the fundamental skills necessary for the provision of spiritual care. However, it has been suggested that it is often difficult to differentiate between essential care and spiritual care. The chapter indicates that nurses may already possess many of the skills necessary to provide spiritual care and what they sometimes lack is confidence in the application of such skills to the spiritual dimension. The chapter suggests that the entire area of spiritual care requires commitment from the nurse and that addressing spiritual needs of patients will be demanding and spiritually exhausting. The importance of having self-awareness to better meet patients' spiritual needs has been stressed. It has been indicated that nurses will only become proficient in attending to patients' spiritual needs if they take a risk and become involved. By providing spiritual care nurses may also attain deeper insights into their own spirituality.

REFERENCES

Burnard P 1987 Spiritual distress and the nursing response: theoretical considerations and counselling skills. Journal of Advanced Nursing 12: 377–382

Burnard P 1988 Discussing spiritual issues with clients. Health Visitor 61
(December): 371–372
Burnard P 1988a The spiritual needs of atheists and agnostics. Professional
Nurse (December): 130–132
Carson V B 1989 Spiritual dimensions of nursing practice. W B Saunders,
Philadelphia
Elsdon M 1995 Spiritual pain in dying people: the nurse's role. Professional
Nurse 10 (10): 641–643
Harrison J 1993 Spirituality and nursing practice. Journal of Clinical Nursing 2:
211–217
Harrison J, Burnard P 1993 Spirituality and nursing practice. Avebury,
Aldershot
Keighley T 1997 Organisational structures and personal spiritual belief.
International Journal of Palliative Nursing 3 (1): 47–51
Leggieri J 1986 Pastoral care in hospital: uniqueness and contribution. Topics in
Clinical Nursing 8 (2): 47–55
McCavery R 1985 Spiritual care in acute illness. In: McGilloway O,
Myco F (eds) Nursing and spiritual care. Harper & Row,
London
McSherry W 1996 Raising the spirits. Nursing Times 92 (3):
48–49
McSherry W 1997 A descriptive survey of nurses' perceptions of
spirituality and spiritual care. Unpublished MPhil thesis, University of
Hull, Hull
Morrison R 1992 Diagnosing pain in patients. Nursing Standard 11 (6):
36–38
Narayanasamy A 1993 Nurses' awareness and educational preparation in
meeting their patients' spiritual needs. Nurse Education Today 13 (3):
196–201
Narayanasamy A 1997 Spiritual dimensions of learning disability. In: Gates B,
Beacock C (eds) Dimensions of learning disability. Baillière Tindall,
London
Ross L A 1997 Nurses' perceptions of spiritual care. Developments in nursing
and health care 13. Avebury, Aldershot
Schoenbeck S L 1994 Called to care: addressing the spiritual needs of patients.
Journal of Practical Nursing (September): 19–23
Speck P 1992 Nursing the soul. Nursing Times 88 (23): 22
Stockwell F 1984 The unpopular patient. Croom Helm, London
Stoter D 1995 Spiritual aspects of health care. Mosby, London
Waugh L A 1992 Spiritual aspects of nursing: a descriptive study of nurses'
perceptions. Unpublished PhD thesis, Queen Margaret College,
Edinburgh

FURTHER READING

*Many books have been written on the subject of counselling and
communication skills in nursing. Such books may have been recommended as
part of a course. With respect to counselling you are advised to consult any of
these texts. The articles and books listed below will consolidate some of the
issues that have been raised in the chapter. Although some of the references
may appear dated, the work of these authors is still relevant and appropriate.*

Burnard P 1987 Spiritual distress and the nursing response: theoretical considerations and counselling skills. Journal of Advanced Nursing 12: 377–382

Burnard P 1988 Discussing spiritual issues with clients. Health Visitor 61(December): 371– 372

McCavery R 1985 Spiritual care in acute illness. In: McGilloway O, Myco F (eds) Nursing and spiritual care. Harper & Row, London

Stoter D 1995 Spiritual aspects of health care. Mosby, London

7

Developments in research and education

INTRODUCTION

Earlier chapters encouraged you to explore the concept of spirituality and the provision of spiritual care with the intention of generating self-awareness. In this chapter we will undertake a brief review of some pioneering research that has been conducted in the USA and the UK concerning spirituality and spiritual care. The research studies presented address both nurses' and patients' perceptions of the spiritual dimension. By reading this chapter you should gain a richer and fuller understanding of how the spiritual dimension is being perceived and developed within nursing practice and education. By critically analysing and reflecting upon the studies you will build on your previous reflections, developing a deeper insight into the terms spirituality and spiritual care as perceived by patients

Activity 7.1

Before proceeding further with this chapter write down anything that you know and understand about the term research.

and nurses. Towards the end of the chapter the growing educational debate that is emerging surrounding spirituality and nurse education is introduced.

In your reflections you have possibly written down a great deal of information concerning your understanding of the term research. The amount of knowledge and insight that you have into research may be dependent upon how much education you received on the subject during your nurse education. The glossary of terms provided (Box 7.1) is designed to give a basic insight so that you can appraise some of the studies that have been undertaken by researchers into the spiritual dimension.

Box 7.1   A brief overview of some of the commonest terminology used in research

Qualitative
　Research that addresses concepts that are very personal and
　　subjective, such as individuals' feelings, thoughts and values.
Quantitative
　Research that is scientific and systematic, generating numerical
　　figures for analysis.
Research process
　A term used to describe the different stages involved in undertaking
　　a research study.
Validity
　Research is said to be valid if it actually achieves the results that it
　　set out to achieve or an instrument measures what it is was
　　supposed to measure.
Reliability
　That a piece of research or instrument can consistently measure or
　　be repeated over time.
Evidence-based care
　A new term that implies that nurses use the most up-to-date
　　research findings to inform nursing practice.
Data
　The information gained while undertaking a piece of research. There
　　are different types of data dependent upon the type of research
　　undertaken – numerical and descriptive.

For further information into any aspect of research you are encouraged to consult one of the many texts that have been written on the subject (see Further reading list at the end of the chapter).

STUDIES EXPLORING NURSES' PERCEPTIONS OF SPIRITUALITY AND SPIRITUAL CARE

A review of the literature suggests that there is a scarcity of research investigating nurses' perceptions of spirituality and spiritual care. Most of the studies undertaken appear to investigate patients' perspectives, with nurses as an adjunct (Conrad 1985, Highfield 1992, Dunn 1993, Emblen & Halstead 1993). Within the last decade a small number of studies have been conducted both in the USA and the UK that have focused primarily upon the nurse. A summary of these studies is provided in Table 7.1. This lack of research into this very important area raises questions about how nurses interpret and provide spiritual care. However, the research that has been undertaken, and published, provides valuable insights. The following section presents some of the research findings, addressing nurses' perceptions of spirituality and spiritual care. The research is presented in chronological order and the contribution and the importance of the research findings is explored.

Caution

The author is very much aware that research into the spiritual dimension is on-going. The research studies presented in this chapter are by no means comprehensive critiques, nor are they exhaustive in that they represent all research undertaken at a given point in time. The purpose of presenting these studies is to demonstrate how the spiritual dimension has been addressed both theoretically and clinically during the last decade. The author has been selective in the studies presented. It must be emphasized that interest in the spiritual dimension is growing within diverse client groups. Therefore the research presented within this chapter is not representative of all research being undertaken or completed within nursing addressing the spiritual dimension.

Table 7.1 Summary of studies addressing nurses' perceptions of spirituality

USA Authors	Date	Area of interest	UK Authors	Date	Area of interest
Highfield & Cason	1983	Spiritual needs of patients: are they recognized?	Waugh	1992	Spiritual aspects of nursing
Boutell & Bozett	1990	Nurses' assessment of patients' spirituality	Harrison & Burnard	1993	Spirituality and nursing practice
Piles	1991	Providing spiritual care	Narayanasamy	1993	Nurses' educational preparedness in meeting patients' spiritual needs
Emblen & Halstead	1993	Spiritual needs and interventions	McSherry	1997	A descriptive survey of nurses' perceptions of spirituality and spiritual care

Nurses' awareness of patients' spiritual concerns

Highfield & Cason (1983) used a descriptive study to identify nurses' awareness of patients' spiritual concerns. The study was conducted using an investigator-designed instrument based around Clinebell's 'religious–existential' framework. Using this instrument, 100 surgical nurses working with oncology patients were surveyed. Of the nurses surveyed, 35 respondents indicated a limited awareness of spiritual needs and problems. Highfield & Cason (1983 p. 191) write:

These results raise some fundamental issues for clinicians, educators, and researchers. Whether or not problems are diagnosed and treated appropriately is the cornerstone of nursing care.

This study highlights a fundamental need for nurses to have some theoretical instruction into the spiritual dimension. The results indicate a need for research to be conducted investigating nurses' perceptions of the concept of spirituality. The inability of the nurses to recognize spiritual needs implies a lack of awareness into what is meant by spirituality and spiritual care. A limitation of this study may well be that the researchers used an instrument that was originally designed for use in pastoral situations. Another limitation is that the study population was small, restricted to 100 surgical nurses working with oncology patients.

Piles (1990) used a survey in an attempt to discover if, or to what extent, spiritual care was being provided to patients manifesting evidence of spiritual needs. A questionnaire was designed based on the research questions and research hypotheses. This was mailed to 300 nurses in four different regions of the USA. Of the 300 questionnaires dispatched only 176 were returned completed, representing a 59% response rate. The questionnaire contained five-point Likert scales, and the results were analysed using multiple regression analysis.

Piles' results indicated that nurses adopted an holistic approach: 95.5% of the nurses surveyed felt that spiritual care was included in holistic care. An interesting finding was that 87.5% of the nurses disagreed that only clergy could provide spiritual care. The results of Piles' research suggested that there was a lack of educational preparedness to meet patients' spiritual needs: 65.9% of the nurses felt inadequately prepared to meet expressed spiritual needs. In relation to practice issues,

87.1% of the nurses indicated time and 70.6% lack of knowledge as being the main obstacles in providing spiritual care.

Piles' survey indicated that there was a willingness for nurses to 'get involved' in the provision of spiritual care. Of the nurses surveyed, 78% agreed that if they had received some educational preparation into spirituality and spiritual care then patients' spiritual need would have been addressed. This willingness is further demonstrated since 89.2% of the nurses surveyed felt that spiritual care should be included in the nursing curricula.

This study has several strengths. First, the survey had a relatively high response rate given the sensitivity of the subject. Second, the results of the data were analysed using advanced statistical methods, which means that the survey could be duplicated, enabling measures of reliability and validity to be further explored. Third, the survey was not localized since it was carried out in four different regions of the USA, suggesting that the results may well reflect national norms.

Activity 7.2

What do you feel about the results of these research findings? Do you think that they have any implications for your practice?

Assessment of spiritual needs

Boutell & Bozett (1990) carried out a survey, using Boutell's inventory for identifying nurses' assessment of patients' spiritual needs, of 817 nurses eligible to practice nursing in Oklahoma, USA. Of these questionnaires 340 (41%) were returned, 29% of which were usable. The inventory contained 76 items divided into two parts. The first collected demographic data, for example gender, age and religious beliefs. The second contained questions addressing assessment of spiritual needs, etc. Answers were obtained using a five-point Likert scale (similar to the one in the Appendix) ranging from 'never' to 'always'. Of the nurses surveyed 34% reported that they assessed their patients' spiritual needs. Boutell's study gained valuable insights into how nurses' perceived spirituality. She identifies that the five components of spirituality commonly assessed by nurses were: fear of medical procedures, patients' sources of inner strength, feelings of hope, religious practices concerned with death, and religious practices concerned with surgery. Boutell suggests that the two least reported aspects of spiritual assessment are integration (spirituality a unifying force) and transcendence (rising above worldly things).

Boutell's work found that age had a significant bearing on whether spiritual needs were assessed. Nurses aged between 50 and 59 were more likely to address spiritual needs than those aged 30–39. The reasoning presented to support these findings was that the older a person becomes, the more likely he or she is to be spiritually aware, since the person may be questioning issues surrounding his or her own mortality and spirituality. A difference was identified in the type of nurse. Psychiatric nurses were more likely to assess a patient's spiritual needs than traditional nurses. This was possibly due to the fact that psychiatric nurses had more time, and they were used to counselling.

In relation to spiritual care and the identification of spiritual needs, 91% of the nurses surveyed obtained information by listening to the patient. Interestingly the least frequently used methods of identifying spiritual needs were discussing with clergy, using the care plan, and asking a significant other. Therefore it would appear that if nurses are to identify and assess a patient's spiritual needs they need time to listen.

This piece of research was restricted in the sense that the response rate was low. One attributing factor may be that the inventory was too long (containing 76 items). However, the research did obtain data that are relevant, identifying how nurses understood the concepts of spirituality and spiritual care. The research was a positive attempt at identifying and quantifying these concepts. The inventory did achieve an alpha coefficient of 0.95, which is an extremely high measure of internal reliability.

Emblen & Halstead (1993) conducted a descriptive qualitative study, using interviews, to collect data to determine how patients, nurses and chaplains defined the phrases 'spiritual needs' and 'spiritual interventions'. Twelve nurses were interviewed. The interviews were transcribed and six categories identified by all three groups as being part of spiritual needs: religious, values, relationships, transcendence, affective feeling

Activity 7.3

Consider the points that have been raised in this book regarding the assessment of spiritual needs. Why do you think nurses may have difficulty in undertaking such assessments? And why is it hard to measure nurses' ability to identify patients' spiritual needs?

and communication. Nursing interventions were identified as prayer, scripture, presence, listening and referral.

A universal approach

Emblen & Halstead's study (1993) is important in that it attempted to gain a cross-section of opinions in how the spiritual dimension is perceived by patients, nurses and chaplains. A serious limitation of the study, identified by the researchers, was that the majority of the respondents had affiliations with one of the standard Western religions: Judaism, Catholicism and Protestantism. This may well explain why the categories highlighted in the research have a religious focus, for example prayer and scripture. Nevertheless, this type of research could be replicated incorporating all patients' and nurses' opinions, not just those within surgical departments.

This need to be more universal in approach is important since surgical departments are usually addressing acute episodes of illness or the disease process. Narayanasamy (1996 p. 412) emphasizes this need for awareness when addressing chronic illness:

Chronic illness may leave a person in a state of spiritual distress which means imbalance or disharmony of mind, body and spirit.

Therefore, if the concept of spirituality is to be thoroughly investigated and understood, it must be investigated by adopting a universal approach, in the sense that it tries to establish a broad understanding of the concept, not just focusing upon specific groups. The results of such specific research may not be representative and generalizable to the larger population.

Waugh (1992), as part of a PhD thesis, conducted an exploratory, descriptive study addressing two research questions: how do nurses perceive spiritual need and spiritual care and try to give the latter in practice; and what factors appear to influence the spiritual care given to patients. The study population consisted of staff nurses and charge nurses working full-time day and night duty on elderly care wards in NHS hospitals in 12 Health Boards in Scotland, a total study population of 1170 nurses. The research instrument, a postal questionnaire, was purposefully designed to meet the needs of the study. Waugh managed to achieve a 67.8% response rate. This response rate is very respectable for a postal survey addressing such a sensitive issue. This high response rate may indicate a shift in nurses' attitudes towards spirituality, suggesting a willingness to enter into a dialogue about the subject.

A summary of the major findings showed that 76.8% of the nurses surveyed stated that they had identified a patient(s) with a spiritual need. An interesting finding was that 55.2% of the nurses surveyed felt that they were more effective than ineffective at meeting these spiritual needs. The nurses surveyed predominately recognized spiritual needs by non-verbal communication. Of the nurses surveyed 34% defined spiritual needs as a need for belief and faith that was mainly concerned with religious aspects of spiritual care; and 51.6% suggested that they would refer on an individual to another person – presumably the hospital chaplain. Despite this finding, 93.7% of the nurses felt that they were directly responsible for providing spiritual care.

Identification of spiritual needs

Waugh identified four factors that were found to be significant in the identification of an individual with a spiritual need. These were: grade, belief system of the nurse, type of ward and geographical location.

Charge nurses were more likely to identify spiritual needs than staff nurses. This finding is surprising given that many charge nurses are now functioning in managerial capacities, and contact with patients is less.

Nurses who had a religious affiliation were more likely to identify spiritual needs.

Nurses working in varied, elderly care wards were more likely to identify spiritual needs than those working on long-term wards.

The locality of the health board appeared to determine whether spiritual needs were identified, although Waugh cannot explain this finding.

In an attempt to explore and explain these factors, Waugh carried out interviews with 12 nurses derived from the study population. These interviews identified four main groups of factors that influenced the spiritual care nurses provided: the patient, other professionals, environment and the nurse.

This qualitative study was a 'milestone' in the investigation of spirituality and spiritual care within the UK. For the first time a large study had been carried out investigating nurses' perceptions of spiritual needs and spiritual care within a large geographical area. Until this study, most of the studies had been on a smaller scale, using interviews. Waugh's study meant that the results of the survey could well be representative and applied to the large population of nursing in Britain. The study generated great insight and provided explanation into how nurses perceived spiritual needs and spiritual care. It provided a foundation for subsequent inquiry.

One limitation of the research originates from the study population – nurses working on care of the elderly wards. The literature suggests that towards the end of life there may well be a revisiting or a return to spiritual values (Carson 1989). If this finding is applied to Waugh's study, then nurses working on wards for the elderly may well be addressing spiritual needs more frequently than those nurses working in more general acute areas.

Harrison & Burnard (1993) in their book *Spirituality and nursing practice* present the findings of a qualitative study into the concept of spirituality, presumed carried out in England. The study used a descriptive, qualitative approach employing in-depth interviews and modified aspects of grounded theory to explore trained nurses' perceptions of the concept of spirituality. The study sought to investigate the concept of spirituality both personally and professionally in order to highlight knowledge and understanding. The study population consisted of ten qualified nurses, working in clinical areas. The length of time individuals had been qualified ranged from 6 months to 3 years. In relation to the study population the researchers felt that it was important to include nurses with whom they had an established relationship of trust and who they felt could articulate their thoughts and feelings clearly.

Several general categories were identified from the interviews. These were then collapsed into three 'higher-order' headings: the concept of spirituality, spirituality and nursing practice, and the spirituality of nurses. Harrison & Burnard discuss in great detail the findings related to the higher-order headings. Summarizing the findings in relation to the concept of spirituality they write (Harrison & Burnard 1993 p. 70):

Generalisations cannot be drawn from these interviews but the varying definitions of spirituality, given by these trained nurses and the case study, do appear to support the literature's recognition of the complexity of spirituality and its unique interpretation by individuals.

When concluding the section addressing spirituality and nursing practice, the authors write (Harrison & Burnard 1993 pp. 84–85):

. . . nurses require more knowledge and greater understanding about spirituality and nursing practice. This has implications for nurse education. Any educational programme about spirituality should carefully consider its content and include such topics as relevance and importance to nursing practice, methods of spiritual assessment and the development of essential skills required for spiritual care.

This study suggests that there is a need for this type of research to be repeated on a sample that is more representative in that a larger and more diverse population of nurses is involved. A limitation of the study is seen in the fact that the sample was purposefully selected, thereby making the findings unrepresentative. However, the study did gain valuable insights into how nurses perceived and addressed the concepts of spirituality and spiritual care within clinical practice. The study indicated that there is still a growing awareness of the importance of the spiritual dimension within nursing in the UK. The study and book are a reference point for subsequent inquiry and debate concerning spirituality and nurse education.

Activity 7.4

Do you think that the research findings emerging from the USA can be representative of how nurses and patients may perceive the concept of spirituality within the UK?

Nurses' perceptions survey

McSherry (1998) presents the findings of a large descriptive survey of nurses of all grades working full- and part-time on wards in a large National Health Service Trust. This work builds upon the work of the aforementioned researchers generating a deeper insight into how nurses perceive spirituality. A questionnaire, with covering letter, was distributed to 1029 nurses. A response rate of 55.3% was obtained, the total number of questionnaires being returned was 559. The questionnaire was designed to gain data that would address the research aims (Box 7.2).

The research identified that nurses perceive spirituality as a universal concept that they feel is relevant to all individuals. Nurses are prepared to participate in the provision of spiritual care, emphasizing the need for a team approach. The nurses surveyed felt that matters concerning the spiritual dimension need to be placed firmly within existing nursing curricula. The abstract, reproduced in Box 7.3, offers a fuller insight into this research. (A copy of the questionnaire used in this study can be found in the Appendix.)

Box 7.2 Research aims

Explore nurses' attitudes to and perceptions of spirituality
Identify whether patients' spiritual needs are being recognized by nurses
Establish whether qualified nurses feel that they are able to meet their patients' spiritual needs
Establish whether qualified nurses feel that they receive sufficient education and training to enable them to meet patients' spiritual needs effectively
Briefly explore the possible associations that may exist between religion and nurses' understanding of spirituality and the provision of spiritual care

Box 7.3   Abstract from the nurses' perception survey (McSherry 1997 pp. 2–3)

This descriptive research investigated Nurses' Perceptions of Spirituality and Spiritual Care, an area of nursing which is very personal, sensitive and shrouded in misconception and ambiguity. The study was designed to address some of these misconceptions by exploring what nurses perceive spirituality to be and how they provide spiritual care. The research was concerned with the identification of patients with spiritual needs, educational issues pertaining to spirituality, and religious practices.

The study was quantitative in design taking the form of a descriptive survey. The Spirituality and Spiritual Care Rating Scale (SSCRS) was specifically designed for this research and was distributed to 1029 Qualified and Unqualified nurses, working on wards in a large National Health Service Trust in East Yorkshire, England. Of the questionnaires distributed 559 were returned, giving a response rate of 55.3%. The SSCRS obtained an alpha coefficient of 0.6443 for the 17-item scale, and when items with low inter-item correlations were removed an alpha coefficient of 0.77 was obtained, indicating an acceptable level of reliability for a newly developed instrument. The questionnaires were analysed using SPSS (Statistical Package for the Social Sciences).

Findings indicated that both qualified (392) 71.4% and unqualified nurses' (68) 12.3% are identifying patients with spiritual needs. Of the qualified nurses who responded (219) 39.9% felt that they were able to meet their patients' spiritual needs. The survey found that patients themselves would indicate to nurses the presence of a spiritual need, (372) 67.8% of the nurses surveyed. These findings demonstrate that nurses are prepared to be involved in the provision of spiritual care. The results raise questions about the quality and type of spiritual care being provided since (290) 52.8% of the qualified nurses stated that they had not received any instruction into the spiritual dimension. The study suggests that nurses have a willingness and desire to know more about the concept. This is evident by the large number of qualified nurses (394) 71.8% who felt that they did not receive sufficient training in this aspect of care. Of the nurses surveyed (421) 76.7% felt that a team approach, (involving the patient, nurses, chaplains, family, friends) was needed in the provision of spiritual care, indicating that nurses felt that no single profession was solely responsible. Religious beliefs and religious practices did not appear to significantly influence the provision of spiritual care. Of the nurses surveyed (409) 74.5% stated that they had a religion but only (160) 29.1% stated that they were practicing their religion.

For the purpose of this study an Exploratory Factor Analysis was used employing Varimax rotation, in an attempt to identify any underlying associations between variables in the SSCRS. This analysis suggested a 15-item instrument with four factor based subscales: Existential Search, Rudiments of Spiritual Care, Universality, Individuality. These factors were described and underlying associations explained in relation to existing literature. The identification of these factors suggests that the nurses surveyed had a broad universal understanding of spirituality, which was relevant to all individuals irrespective of religious affiliation. The findings also indicate that nurses are aware that the provision of spiritual care is inherently different to the provision of general care.

The findings of this research validates previous British studies addressing this aspect of care (Simsen, 1985, Waugh, 1992, Narayanasamy, 1993, Harrison & Burnard, 1993). This process of validation suggests that these results may well reflect the larger population of nurses. However caution needs to be exercised in that the SSCRS is a newly developed instrument which will need to be refined and validated by subsequent research.

Summary of the main research findings and limitations

The studies reviewed investigating nurses' perceptions of spirituality and spiritual care demonstrate that there is still a fundamental need to establish how nurses *interpret* and *define* spirituality and spiritual care. The studies previously undertaken have developed some insight and understanding of spiritual needs and spiritual care, yet there is an apparent lack of research focusing primarily upon the concept of spirituality in the broader sense. The studies have focused upon the nurses' ability to define and meet spiritual needs, and upon the provision of spiritual care. They have targeted specific populations of nurses such as nurses working in oncology and surgical units or nurses working in care of the elderly wards. There is a need to investigate nurses working within *all specialties*, irrespective of grade, in order to gain a wider understanding of nurses' perceptions of spirituality and spiritual care. By extending the boundaries of investigation a more comprehensive picture of how nurses perceive the spiritual dimension will be obtained.

STUDIES EXPLORING PATIENTS' PERCEPTIONS OF SPIRITUALITY AND SPIRITUAL CARE

This section will explore some of the research that has been conducted in the USA and the UK focusing upon patients' perceptions of spirituality. Again this is not a definitive list of all the research available nor has a detailed appraisal of the research been offered. Table 7.2 provides a brief summary of some of the authors and the areas of spirituality investigated.

Table 7.2 A summary of some studies addressing patients' perceptions of spirituality

USA Authors	Date	Area of interest	UK Authors	Date	Area of interest
Stallwood	1967	Spiritual needs survey	Simsen	1985	Spiritual needs in illness and hospitalization
Martin et al	1976	Spiritual needs of patients study	Ross (née Waugh)	1997	Elderly patients' perceptions of their spiritual needs and care: a pilot study
Soderstrom & Martinson	1987	Patients' spiritual coping strategies; nurse and patient perspectives			In comparison to the number of studies conducted in the USA it is apparent that there is a scarcity of published literature addressing aspects of spirituality in relation to patients, clients or users of health care in the UK
Soeken & Carson	1987	Responding to the spiritual needs of the chronically ill			The author is aware that there are some excellent undergraduate dissertations and postgraduate theses that have been conducted by nurses in the UK
Reed	1991	Preferences for spirituality related nursing interventions among terminally ill and non-terminally ill hospitalized adults and well adults			Other members of the multidisciplinary team, in particular chaplains, have also conducted research

NB: Many of the above authors have undertaken further research and contributed substantially in this dimension of nursing.

Patients' awareness of spiritual needs

Stallwood (1969) conducted a spiritual needs survey, supported by The Nurses Christian Fellowship, to determine patients' awareness of their spiritual needs. A bias that may have entered this study could be due to the study being sponsored by a Christian organization. The study involved interviewing 109 patients in hospitals and extended care facilities in various parts of the USA. The results of this descriptive study suggest that patients are able to recognize their own spiritual needs and do have a definite understanding of the concept that has purpose and meaning for them. The patients expressed a need for assistance in meeting these spiritual needs not only from the hospital chaplain, minister, priest or rabbi, but also from the nurses who cared for them. This study is unique in that it was the first of its kind, and it demonstrated that patients did find meaning and purpose in the spiritual dimension that enabled them to cope with hospitalization.

A valid point that emerges from Stallwood's study is that its methodology embraced a cross-sectional design, addressing the spiritual needs of both sexes, young and old (18 years–90 years) who were in either medical or surgical specialties. One could argue that this study sought to investigate the spiritual needs of patients in acute illness. A major limitation of this study, which has already been identified by Kearney (1994), is that it is now long out of date (it is 25 years old). Therefore, the study will probably not reflect the current changes in thought and attitudes surrounding spirituality in today's modernistic and secular society.

Martin et al (1976), sponsored by The Nurses Christian Fellowship, performed an empirical descriptive study exploring the spiritual needs of patients using survey methods by designing and administering two instruments for data collection, a questionnaire and an interview schedule. A sample of 90 adults within two general hospitals was obtained. The purpose of this study was to determine what spiritual needs hospitalized persons experience, what nursing actions help resolve these needs, and how patients feel about receiving spiritual care from a nurse.

The results of Martin's study confirmed and validated Stallwood's earlier work. The research revealed that spiritual needs were identified by both sexes, females being able to verbalize their spiritual needs more easily than males. The clergy were identified as the patients' main preference for discussing spiritual matters. The patients identified four important spiritual needs: relief from fear of death; a knowledge of God's presence; a need to feel supported and cared for by another person; and receiving the sacraments. The last spiritual need is probably due to the fact that 90% of the study population were of the Catholic (48%) and Protestant (42%) churches that attach great importance to the sacraments. The study also highlighted that patients appreciated the concern and kindness shown by nurses expressing a desire to be allowed to talk to and to be listened to by nurses more closely. These findings demonstrate that patients are familiar with and able to identify their own spiritual needs. They present an argument for improved nurse education and knowledge concerning spirituality so that nurses can offer more assistance and support to patients during periods of hospitalization.

A major limitation of the study is that it does not adequately represent the spiritual needs of the atheist or agnostic, who accounted for only 8% of the study population. This study, like Stallwood's (1969), appears to have a Judeo–Christian bias or focus. Perhaps this could be due to the geographical or demographic location of the studies, which are not mentioned. One must also bear in mind that both studies were supported by The Nurses Christian Fellowship of America, which may have biased the results (Kearney 1994).

Activity 7.5

In your experience do you think that if you asked patients the question 'Do you have any spiritual needs?' they would understand what you were asking?

Coping strategies

Sodestrom & Martinson (1987) carried out a descriptive study in an attempt to describe the spiritual coping strategies of 25 hospitalized patients with cancer and their nurses' awareness of these strategies. A convenience sample of 25 nurses working in an oncology unit in a major non-sectarian medical centre were paired with 25 patients. The researchers used interviews in order to obtain information into any spiritual coping strategies patients used to deal with cancer. The results revealed that 88% of patients used a variety of spiritual activities and resource people while coping with cancer. Of the patients interviewed 66% reported an increase in awareness and practice of their spiritual beliefs since diagnosis. The findings showed that nurses had difficulty identifying patients' use of spiritual coping strategies. This is not surprising since 56% of the nurses interviewed had difficulty in identifying the patients' religions. This raises questions about the initial admission procedure and its reliability. Forbis (1988 p. 159) states:

the admission interview should include questions related to religious affiliation.

This piece of research validates the theories that illness and disease can challenge a patient's belief system, causing a refocusing upon the spiritual dimension. The results demonstrate a positive relationship between spirituality and coping. The research draws attention to a major discrepancy in the nurse's lack of knowledge, awareness, and ability to support patients who are forced to evaluate the meaning of suffering and death since the majority of patients in this study (92%) were terminally ill with a prognosis of less than 6 months. These results are quite alarming when one considers that the patients interviewed sensed an increased awareness of the spiritual dimension and the nurses looking after them were on a specialist oncology unit.

Patients' spiritual needs and resources

All of the previous research studies investigating patients' perceptions and attitudes towards spirituality discussed above were conducted in the USA. The first British study investigating the spiritual needs and resources of patients was conducted by Simsen (1985). The results revealed that patients had a constant need to make sense of their circumstances and to find meaning in the events of their everyday relationships and life. Simsen used a qualitative design, interviewing a sample of 45 male and female surgical and medical patients who had a diverse range of cultural and religious beliefs.

Activity 7.6 Searching the database

If you have access to a library that offers facilities to do a simple literature search, type in the words 'spirituality' or 'spiritual care' and review the results. Ask yourself what the results suggest about this aspect of nursing.

The research findings demonstrated that patients do find value and meaning in the spiritual dimension and that they are willing to discuss matters that are sensitive and personal. Simsen also highlighted that personal beliefs and practices are sometimes rated higher than the institutional forms. Due to the small study sample the results cannot be generalized. Nevertheless, Simsen's study is a milestone in the investigation of spirituality within the UK because it was the first of its kind. Simsen's efforts attempted and succeeded in breaking the taboos, barriers and misconceptions associated with the concept of spirituality by British nurses. Her study has set a precedent that is now gaining momentum, inspiring more British research and interest.

Spirituality-related nursing interventions

The previous studies investigating patients' attitudes and perceptions surrounding the concept of spirituality have been descriptive, exploring and clarifying understanding and definition of the concept. Reed (1991) conducted research attempting to determine terminally ill and non-terminally ill hospitalized patients' preference for spirituality-related nursing interventions, attempting to identifying differences between the groups. The study population consisted of 300 adults: 100 had an incurable cancer; 100 did not have a serious illness; 100 were non-hospitalized healthy people taken from the local community. A questionnaire format was used to gather the data. Participants within this study identified several interventions for spiritual needs that can be included under the heading of nursing practice such as arranging visits from the clergy; creating an environment that will enable patients to fulfil their own spiritual practices (allowing solitude for prayer or private devotions); simply talking and listening to the patient; and involving family in spiritual activities.

These are all interventions that can be facilitated by nurses in the management of spiritual needs. The differences found between the groups of patients emphasized the need for care to be individualized, patient-centred and specific. Owing to their poor physical condition and mobility, the terminally ill found it difficult to participate in structured religious practices. The nursing staff therefore had to facilitate by preparing the patients' environment, allowing time for quiet reflection and private spiritual practices. The need for good communication and patient interaction was ranked highly by the terminally ill in their choice of interventions. The non-terminally ill and non-hospitalized groups expressed a need to participate in structured religious practices and to attend chapel.

The findings of this study emphasize the need for nurses to be sensitive to the spiritual needs of all patients. The results demonstrate that all categories of patients are able to identify and order spiritually-related nursing intervention. The order of these interventions can be determined by the nature of the illness or reason for hospitalization. The results highlight a need for a multidisciplinary team approach to meeting spiritual needs since 'arrange a visit with clergy' was the spiritual intervention most frequently identified by all three groups. This cross-sectional study has its limitations, which Reed acknowledges, for example the use of an open-ended question as a seventh response choice rather than as a primary question. Nevertheless, the results are significant and relevant because they present the patients' ability to assess spiritual interventions. The research attempted to relate the concept of spirituality directly and professionally to nursing practice. Reed has tried to validate clinical experiences highlighting some of the inconsistencies that exist between empirical and clinical knowledge. The research suggests a change of focus in addressing the spiritual dimension from clarification and explanation to application in clinical practice.

Assessing spiritual health

Highfield (1992) conducted a descriptive, cross-sectional survey designed to investigate the spiritual health of oncology patients and to see how effectively oncology nurses assessed spiritual health. Spiritual health inventories were distributed to a convenient sample of nurse and patient pairs within two hospitals. The results showed that the nurses were unable to assess their patients' spiritual health status accurately. The nurses and the patient subjects preferred different spiritual caregivers, despite both groups ranking family member or friend number one.

Highfield attempts to measure systematically the effectiveness of the nurses' ability to assess patients' spiritual health status accurately. The study attempts to investigate the nurses' theoretical and practical understanding of patients' spiritual health. Yet there exist possible explanations that could account for the nurses' inability to assess spiritual health status accurately. The short period of time that the primary nurse had to establish a trusting, meaningful and therapeutic relationship with the patient could be one reason. The majority of the nurses in the study had only cared for the patient for between 1 and 2 days. Although a possible 7 hours each day could have been spent on nurse–patient interaction, that is unlikely because the nurse's time will have been spent on other tasks and duties. Therefore the possibility exists that the nurse may not have known the patient thoroughly. The nature of spirituality being very sensitive and personal suggests that the male patients in this study (70%) felt inhibited, not disclosing valuable information regarding spiritual needs and thus distorting the assessment. These gender differences, highlighted by Martin et al's (1976) earlier work, may therefore have distorted the results. The results of Highfield's study cannot be generalized since they reflect only one category of patient – oncology – and the number of possible variables that appear to distort the research findings need clarifying and investigating further.

Comparing perspectives

After surveying the literature, Emblen & Halstead (1993) discovered that no studies had been undertaken to compare the spiritual perspectives of patients with that of nurses and chaplains. In order to address this discrepancy the researchers conducted a descriptive (qualitative) study to collect interview data to determine how patients, nurses and chaplains are defining spiritual needs and spiritual intervention. The population consisted of 19 surgical patients, 12 nurses and 7 chaplains. The interview results were categorized, itemized and classified according to six categories: religious, values, relationships, transcendence, affective feeling and communication. The participants identified five nursing interventions: prayer, scripture, presence, listening, and referral. Martin et al (1976) and Reed (1991) highlighted the majority of these interventions. The results demonstrated the need for nurses and chaplains to work in collaboration. The findings stress the importance of nurses having the ability to perform comprehensive spiritual needs assessment, probably incorporating the six categories identified.

The study was limited by the category of patient (surgical), age and religious orientation. The study was therefore restricted by only including one category of patient. If one views spiritual development along a lifespan continuum, then the spiritual needs of people differ at certain stages in the development process (Carson 1989). The mean age of the patients in this study was 54 years – middle life. Perhaps younger or older patients might have given different perspectives. The authors state that the most serious limitation is that the majority of respondents identified with one of the standard Western religions, introducing a Judeo–Christian bias.

Summary of the main research findings and limitations

These research studies indicate that patients do have a personal, deep understanding and awareness of the spiritual dimension, an awareness that is often acutely developed and increased in times of illness or personal crisis. Despite the sensitive and personal nature of the subject patients display a willingness to talk openly about their understanding, reflections upon and attitudes surrounding spirituality. The studies presented are comprehensive, presenting a cross-sectional analysis of the spiritual dimension as perceived by the patient. Nevertheless, there are still many patient perspectives left uncovered. All the studies excluded patients under the age of 18 years, probably due to legal and ethical considerations. This point is extremely important since it indicates that there are certain diverse client groups that are neglected in research addressing spirituality such as children and individuals with learning disabilities. The literature

Activity 7.7

Do you think spirituality helps patients cope with their illness or condition? Can you think of any cases from your own practice that might confirm the research presented in this section?

review reveals that there is a scarcity of research conducted within the UK concentrating on patients' perspectives of spirituality or the use of spirituality in coping with illness or disease.

SPIRITUALITY AND NURSE EDUCATION

This section introduces the educational issues surrounding the concept of spirituality, exploring how and if it should be taught within programmes of nurse education. Several of the research studies mentioned earlier in this chapter have indicated a fundamental need for spirituality to be formally integrated within programmes of nurse education. This need has been recognized and addressed within the USA, but within the UK the process of integration has been extremely slow despite nurse researchers and educationalists drawing attention to this omission within existing nurse curricula.

During the course of your nurse training you may or may not have received any formal education into the spiritual dimension. McSherry's (1997) research indicated that some nurses received educational instruction while others received limited instruction surrounding religious practices or a talk from the hospital chaplain. At present within the UK there is no uniform policy that states spirituality should be taught, nor are there any guidelines on what or how it should be taught. It would

Activity 7.8

Spend several minutes reflecting upon your own nurse education. This could be either pre-registration or education undertaken as part of your continuing professional development. Write down any education that you received that addressed the subject of spirituality or spiritual care.

appear that the teaching of spirituality is very much left to the devices of individual institutions or educationalists who have an interest in the subject. Ironically the competency statements that nurses should achieve for registration state that a student nurse should be able to assess, plan, implement and evaluate spiritual care (UKCC 1986). The dilemma is how students, or indeed any nurses, are to provide spiritual care if they do not receive some form of educational preparation that may generate insight and self-awareness.

Emerging debates

Bradshaw (1997) suggests a need for caution in relation to the teaching of spirituality in that the concept is not something that can be taught by theoretical or experiential analysis but rather spiritual awareness comes about through clinical experience and exposure. The growing debate is whether spirituality should be 'taught' or is it something that is 'caught' in practice? Bradshaw warns that the danger of teaching about spirituality is that it becomes another component that is added into nursing curricula, thus fragmenting the individual and defeating the notion of holistic care.

If spirituality is not taught by traditional methods and it is left to be caught by nurses in practice, then there is the danger that spiritual awareness may not be generated or developed. The process of socialization and skill acquisition that is dependent upon supervision and exposure in practice may result in patients' spiritual needs not being addressed by nurses in practice. The problem with acquiring skills through exposure and experience may mean that neophyte nurses model and shape their practice by observing and imitating the behaviours and practices displayed by their superiors. If such role models do not address the spiritual dimension of their patients, then this

Activity 7.9

Spend several minutes reflecting upon the emerging debates, writing down what you feel are the pros and cons of both sides. Can you think of any solutions that may be a way forward?

could result in the cycle being perpetuated and patients' spiritual needs will constantly be neglected. However, if neophyte nurses have some insight into the spiritual dimension they will be able to recognize a spiritual need when it arises, and they will possibly address the perceived need despite the inherent pressures of going against the grain. To illustrate this point, think of an occasion(s) when as a student nurse or a neophyte nurse in practice you were given instruction into the spiritual dimension, or can you recall when you last observed your mentor or preceptor provide an aspect of spiritual care? Bradshaw's concerns are justified in that she does not want to see spirituality as something of an amendment or an addition to the individual, but rather as a set of characteristics that is acquired through exposure in practice, as occurred in the 'old' apprenticeship style of training.

Formal integration

During the late 1980s and early 1990s nurse educationalists in the UK have campaigned relentlessly for the formal integration of the subject within programmes of nurse education (Burnard 1990, Harrison & Burnard 1993, Narayanasamy 1993, Ross 1996, McSherry & Draper 1997). Ross (1996 p. 43) writes:

Guidelines for nurse education stress the need to teach spiritual care to nurses but it is not clear how the subject should be taught or how effective any teaching is in helping nurses to give spiritual care.

This quotation supports previous claims for formal integration while highlighting a need for guidelines on how this might be achieved from nursing professional bodies.

There is a need for nurse educationalists to take a step back and review the situation in the light of all the evidence and debates that are developing. The process of integration may not be that simple because there are several barriers that must be considered in any curriculum innovation (McSherry & Draper 1997). One major barrier is that curriculum review is often slow and it is hard to balance the content of the curriculum. If something is to be added then often it means something else has to be shortened or removed.

However, over a decade ago Carson & Gerardi (1985) introduced a course called 'Spirituality in Nursing Practice' within a nursing faculty in a secular university in America with relatively good success and positive evaluations from students. Similarly within the UK individuals with a keen interest have undertaken similar innovations designing modules, workshops, study days and conferences in order to generate awareness of the importance of spirituality within health care. These innovations and labours would be strengthened if there were consistency and unity, i.e. some form of central control indicating content, methods, and importantly assessment of what should and should not be taught, instead of leaving it to an ad hoc basis. Yet some insight and education is probably better than none at all.

Teaching methods

Bradshaw (1996) is right in that spirituality as a subject is deeply personal, sensitive and highly subjective. Because of this most of the issues associated with the subject do not lend themselves to many of the formal methods of classroom teaching.

Several nurse educationalists have offered suggestions as to the methods that may be suitable for the exploration of the spiritual dimension by nurses (Burnard 1988, Harrison 1993, Bush 1999). It would appear that an important factor is the fostering of a teaching environment that is safe and confidential where students or delegates can explore spiritual issues feeling supported and secure. One of the major concerns with the introduction of Project 2000 was the large increase in student numbers associated with intakes of between 30 and 100 students. Some subjects by their very nature can be addressed in the confines of a lecture and delivered to large audiences. However, matters surrounding spirituality are best delivered in groups of between 6 and 15. Any larger size makes facilitation difficult for the teacher.

Activity 7.10

Spend several minutes reflecting upon your own educational experiences – how do you feel spirituality should be taught to nurses? Which type of teaching methods do you think may assist nurses in acquiring these skills and knowledge?

Throughout this book many situations have been presented that have asked for reflection – generating insight into one's own feelings and attitudes towards a specific matter. These workshop activities appear to generate discussion and debate when addressing matters concerning spirituality within the classroom. Therefore group work, reflection and exercises that generate self-awareness are more suitable for exploring the personal, sensitive and subjective aspects of spirituality. The didactic nature of formal lectures makes them unsuitable for addressing the spiritual dimension.

Duration

The length of time spent addressing matters concerning spirituality must be considered. It is totally unrealistic to think that everything there is to know about spirituality and the provision

---

Box 7.4 Outline of a 2-day course, 'Introduction to the spiritual dimensions of nursing practice'

Day 1

09.30–11.00	Introduction
	Outline of the two days
	Introductory task (Task A)
11.00–11.20	Break (refreshments available)
11.20–12.30	Group work – Using case studies (Task B)
12.30–13.00	Recap of morning session
13.00–14.00	Lunch
14.00–15.00	Spirituality: an exploration of the concept
15.00–15.20	Break (refreshments available)
15.20–16.20	Skills required by nurses to address spiritual needs (a counselling approach)
16.20–16.30	Evaluation of Day 1

Day 2

09.30–11.00	Spirituality and the nursing process (practical session using case studies)
11.00–11.20	Break (refreshments available)
11.20–12.40	Feedback from group exercise: look at barriers that prevent nurses from implementing spiritual care
12.40–13.00	Recap of morning session
13.00–14.00	Lunch
14.00–15.00	An exploration of some of the institutional religions
15.00–15.20	Break (refreshments available)
15.20–16.20	Support networks (discussion)
16.20–16.30	Evaluation of Day 2

of spiritual care can be presented in sufficient depth in a 2- or 3-hour lecture. Therefore when considering the formal integration of spirituality into existing nursing curricula this important issue must be raised (Box 7.4 presents the outline of a 2-day course addressing spirituality and spiritual care). Spirituality may be addressed within the confines of a single module or be revisited throughout the 3-year training programme as a major theme that is revisited within the boundaries of different modules such as nursing theory, communication skills, legal and ethical, multicultural issues or death and dying. Adopting this approach would help alleviate some of the concerns that spirituality is seen as an afterthought.

Facilitator

The question of who should teach matters associated with spirituality is another point that must be considered in depth. In the past spirituality was usually addressed by an hour or two in the company of the hospital chaplain. However, in a changing educational climate and in a society that is sometimes sceptical of formal religious practice how feasible is it to rely solely upon the hospital chaplain? Yet many hospital chaplains are ecumenical in that they provide pastoral and spiritual support to individuals from a range of religious affiliations. Perhaps a way forward is to introduce a team approach to the teaching of the spiritual dimension. It must be emphasized that the teaching of matters surrounding spirituality is very demanding and tiring in that it places a great demand on the emotional and psychological reserve of the teacher. The individuals who teach the subject must have an awareness and a degree of acceptance with their own spirituality in order to offer support to others. The notion of team teaching helps to reduce the emotional demands placed upon one individual while drawing upon the expertise of another.

CONCLUSION

This chapter has introduced you to aspects of the spiritual dimension that have been investigated by nurse researchers. The results generated indicate that spirituality is recognized and fundamental to individuals' health and sense of well-being.

The studies provide a deeper insight into how nurses and patients perceive the concepts of spirituality and spiritual care. As more research is undertaken evidence is emerging that will inform and develop nursing practice, leading to improvements in the quality of spiritual care provided. As more research is undertaken into the spiritual dimension and 'old' research disseminated and evaluated, this should directly influence the way that spirituality is addressed within nurse education. The fact that individuals are generating debate and discussion that is international is positive. The wheels of change are slow but through perseverance and research the spiritual dimension will remain a focus of enquiry within the nursing profession.

Final thought

Spend some time reflecting upon the main findings of the studies that have been presented in this chapter and write down what implications they have for you in the way that spiritual care is provided by you or your colleagues.

REFERENCES

Boutell K A, Bozett F W 1990 Nurses' assessment of patients' spirituality: continuing education implications. Journal of Continuing Education in Nursing 21 (4): 172–176

Bradshaw A 1996 The legacy of Nightingale. Nursing Times 92 (6): 42–43

Bradshaw A 1997 Teaching spiritual care to nurses: an alternative approach. International Journal of Palliative Nursing 3 (1): 51–57

Burnard P 1988 Searching for meaning. Nursing Times 84 (37): 34, 36

Burnard P 1990 Learning to care for the spirit. Nursing Standard 4 (18): 38–39

Bush T 1999 Journalling and the teaching of spirituality. Nurse Education Today 19: 20–28

Carson V B 1989 Spiritual dimensions of nursing practice. W B Saunders, Philadelphia

Carson V, Gerardi R 1985 Spirituality for credit: finding a place in the secular curriculum. Journal of Christian Nursing 2 (3): 28–30

Conrad N L 1985 Spiritual support for the dying. Nursing Clinics of North America 20 (2): 415–426

Dunn P M 1993 An investigation into the concept of spiritual needs of hospitalised patients, from a nursing perspective. Unpublished dissertation, Institute of Nursing Studies, University of Hull, Hull

Emblen J D, Halstead L 1993 Spiritual needs and interventions: comparing the views of patients, nurses and chaplains. Clinical Nurse Specialist 7 (4): 175–182

Forbis P A 1988 Meeting patients' spiritual needs. Geriatric Nursing 9 (3): 158–159

Harrison J 1993 Spirituality and nursing practice. Journal of Clinical Nursing 2: 211–217

Harrison J, Burnard P 1993 Spirituality and nursing practice. Avebury, Aldershot

Highfield M F 1992 Spiritual health of oncology patients: nurse and patient perspectives. Cancer Nursing 15 (1): 1–8

Highfield M F, Cason C 1983 Spiritual needs of patients: are they recognised? Cancer Nursing (June): 187–192

Kearney S 1994 Spirituality as a coping mechanism in multiple sclerosis: the patient's perspective. Unpublished dissertation, Institute of Nursing Studies, University of Hull, Hull

Martin C, Burrows C, Pomilio J 1976 Spiritual needs of patients. In: Shelly J A, Fish S (1988) Spiritual care: the nurse's role, 3rd edn. Inter Varsity Press, Illinois

McSherry W 1997 A descriptive survey of nurses' perceptions of spirituality and spiritual care. Unpublished MPhil thesis, University of Hull, Hull

McSherry W 1998 Nurses' perceptions of spirituality and spiritual care. Nursing Standard 13 (4): 36–40

McSherry W, Draper P 1997 The spiritual dimension: why the absence within nursing curricula? Nurse Education Today 17: 413–417

Narayanasamy A 1993 Nurses' awareness and educational preparation in meeting their patients' spiritual needs. Nurse Education Today 13 (3): 196–201

Narayanasamy A 1996 Spiritual care of chronically ill patients. British Journal of Nursing 5 (7): 411–416

Piles C (1990) Providing spiritual care. Nurse Educator 15 (1): 36–41

Reed P R 1991 Preferences for spirituality related nursing interventions among terminally ill and non-terminally ill hospitalised adults and well adults. Applied Nursing Research 4 (3): 122–128

Ross L A 1996 Teaching spiritual care to nurses. Nurse Education Today 16: 38–43

Ross L A 1997 Elderly patients' perceptions of their spiritual needs and care: a pilot study. Journal of Advanced Nursing 26: 710–715

Simsen B 1985 Spiritual needs and resources in illness and hospitalisation. Unpublished MSc thesis, University of Manchester, Manchester

Sodestrom K E, Martinson I M 1987 Patients' spiritual coping strategies: a study of nurse and patient perspectives. Oncology Nursing Forum 14 (2): 41–46

Soeken K L, Carson V J 1987 Responding to the spiritual needs of the chronically ill. Nursing Clinics of North America 22 (3): 603–611

Stallwood J 1969 Spiritual needs survey. In: Shelly J A, Fish S (eds) 1988 Spiritual care: the nurse's role, 3rd edn. Inter Varsity Press, Illinois

United Kingdom Central Council for Nursing, Midwifery and Health Visiting 1986 Project 2000 – a new preparation for practice. UKCC, London

Waugh L A 1992 Spiritual aspects of nursing: a descriptive study of nurses' perceptions. Unpublished PhD thesis, Queen Margaret College, Edinburgh

FURTHER READING

Research texts
Any of these texts will provide the reader with a detailed insight into the different approaches to research and the stages involved in the research process.

Burns N and Grove S K 1987 The practice of nursing research conduct, critique and utilisation. W B Saunders, Philadelphia

Cormack D F S 1991 The research process in nursing, 2nd edn. Blackwell Scientific Publications, Oxford

Talbot L 1995 Principles and practice of nursing research. Mosby, London

Research studies addressing nurses' perceptions of spirituality
The following texts will bring the reader up to date with the state of research addressing spirituality within the UK. The reader is also encouraged to look at other international studies that have been referenced throughout the chapter for a more global appreciation.

McSherry W 1998 Nurses' perceptions of spirituality and spiritual care. Nursing Standard 13 (4): 36–40

Ross L A 1997 Elderly patients' perceptions of their spiritual needs and care: a pilot study. Journal of Advanced Nursing 26: 710–715

Ross L A 1997 Nurses' perceptions of spiritual care. Avebury, Aldershot

Waugh L A 1992 Spiritual aspects of nursing: a descriptive study of nurses' perceptions. Unpublished PhD thesis, Queen Margaret College, Edinburgh

Research studies addressing patients' perceptions of spirituality

Simsen B (1985) Spiritual needs and resources in illness and hospitalisation. Unpublished MSc thesis, University of Manchester, Manchester

Spirituality and education
The following texts will bring the reader up to date with the growing debate addressing spirituality within nurse education in the UK. The reader is also encouraged to look at other international studies that have been referenced throughout the chapter for a more global appreciation.

Bradshaw A 1997 Teaching spiritual care to nurses: an alternative approach. International Journal of Palliative Nursing 3 (1): 51–57

Burnard P 1990 Learning to care for the spirit. Nursing Standard 4 (18): 38–39

McSherry W, Draper P 1997 The spiritual dimension: why the absence within nursing curricula? Nurse Education Today 17: 413–417

Narayanasamy A 1993 Nurses' awareness and educational preparation in meeting their patients' spiritual needs. Nurse Education Today 13 (3): 196–201

Ross L A 1996 Teaching spiritual care to nurses. Nurse Education Today 16: 38–43

Appendix

Appendix: Spirituality and spiritual care rating scale

INTRODUCTION

Research into spirituality is discussed in detail in Chapter 7. The rating scale used by McSherry (1997) is described below, and the text of the questionnaire used to provide a spirituality and spiritual care rating scale (SSCRS) is reproduced in full.

NOTES ON CONSTRUCTION

As you are aware, the concept of spirituality is very broad and subjective. Therefore, if an individual respondent were simply asked to write down what he or she thought spirituality was, some might well be able to write a thesis. To prevent this and to make statistical analysis easier, the rating scale was devised and constructed covering key areas associated with spirituality and spiritual care. The material for these questions was identified in the literature. Questions were then formulated and constructed.

Box A.1   Fundamental areas pertaining to spirituality

(1) Hope
(2) Meaning and purpose
(3) Forgiveness
(4) Beliefs and values
(5) Spiritual care
(6) Relationships
(7) Belief in a God or deity
(8) Morality
(9) Creativity and self-expression

Box A.2 Scoring for the scale

1 = Strongly disagree
2 = Disagree
3 = Uncertain
4 = Agree
5 = Strongly agree

The 23-item scale was structured around nine fundamental areas pertaining to spirituality that have been documented or identified in the literature by several authors (Frankl 1987, Shelly & Fish 1988, Carson 1989, Narayanasamy 1991, Waugh 1992, Emblen & Halstead 1993, Harrison & Burnard 1993). It was around the work of these key authors that the framework for the SSCRS was designed and structured.

The rating scale was constructed using a five-point Likert scale. A five-point scale was chosen because more complex scoring methods had been shown to possess no advantage (Oppenheim 1992 p. 195). Respondents were asked to circle their preferred answer. Scoring was as described in Box A.2.

Originally a 23-item pool was formulated. In the first draft the Ethics Committee felt that the items seemed to follow on from each other in sequence – a response-set bias. In order to address this possible response set the 17 items used in the final rating scale were randomized using random number tables and individualized. This meant that each item began with 'I believe spirituality . . .' or 'I believe nurses can provide spiritual care by . . .'. In order to prevent any response-set bias, 25% of the 23 items were phrased in the negative, i.e. 'I believe spirituality is not concerned with a belief and faith in a God or supreme being'. These measures taken to prevent a response-set bias appeared to be effective. When the 23 items were analysed after the pre-pilot phases six items were found not to be contributing to the overall scores in a significant way; these were removed from the item pool. Originally the SSCRS was designed in two parts: questions a–q addressed elements of spirituality and questions r–w addressed issues pertaining to spiritual care. Eventually all the questions in the scale were randomized and integrated. Integrating questions was another measure taken to try and prevent any response-set bias.

It is anticipated that the SSCRS can be used by researchers investigating the spiritual dimension.

SPIRITUALITY AND SPIRITUAL CARE RATING SCALE (SSCRS)

For each question please *circle* one answer that best reflects the extent to which you agree or disagree with each statement.

a) I believe nurses can provide spiritual care by arranging a visit by the hospital chaplain or the patient's own religious leader if requested

Strongly disagree   *Disagree*   *Uncertain*   *Agree*   *Strongly agree*
   *   *   *   *   *

b) I believe nurses can provide spiritual care by showing kindness, concern and cheerfulness when giving care

Strongly disagree   *Disagree*   *Uncertain*   *Agree*   *Strongly agree*
   *   *   *   *   *

c) I believe spirituality is concerned with a need to forgive and a need to be forgiven

Strongly disagree   *Disagree*   *Uncertain*   *Agree*   *Strongly agree*
   *   *   *   *   *

d) I believe spirituality involves only going to church/place of worship

Strongly disagree   *Disagree*   *Uncertain*   *Agree*   *Strongly agree*
   *   *   *   *   *

e) I believe spirituality is not concerned with a belief and faith in a God or Supreme Being

Strongly disagree   *Disagree*   *Uncertain*   *Agree*   *Strongly agree*
   *   *   *   *   *

f) I believe spirituality is about finding meaning in the good and bad events of life

Strongly disagree   Disagree   Uncertain   Agree   Strongly agree
*   *   *   *   *

g) I believe nurses can provide spiritual care by spending time with a patient giving support and reassurance especially in time of need

Strongly disagree   Disagree   Uncertain   Agree   Strongly agree
*   *   *   *   *

h) I believe nurses can provide spiritual care by enabling a patient to find meaning and purpose in his or her illness

Strongly disagree   Disagree   Uncertain   Agree   Strongly agree
*   *   *   *   *

i) I believe spirituality is about having a sense of hope in life

Strongly disagree   Disagree   Uncertain   Agree   Strongly agree
*   *   *   *   *

j) I believe spirituality is to do with the way one conducts one's life here and now

Strongly disagree   Disagree   Uncertain   Agree   Strongly agree
*   *   *   *   *

k) I believe nurses can provide spiritual care by listening to and allowing patients time to discuss and explore their fears, anxieties and troubles

Strongly disagree   Disagree   Uncertain   Agree   Strongly agree
*   *   *   *   *

l) I believe spirituality is a unifying force which enables one to be at peace with oneself and the world

Strongly disagree   Disagree   Uncertain   Agree   Strongly agree
*   *   *   *   *

m) I believe spirituality does not include areas such as art, creativity and self-expression

Strongly disagree   Disagree   Uncertain   Agree   Strongly agree
*   *   *   *   *

n) I believe nurses can provide spiritual care by having respect for privacy, dignity and religious and cultural beliefs of a patient

Strongly disagree   *Disagree*   *Uncertain*   *Agree*   *Strongly agree*
        *   *   *   *   *

o) I believe spirituality involves personal friendships and relationships

Strongly disagree   *Disagree*   *Uncertain*   *Agree*   *Strongly agree*
        *   *   *   *   *

p) I believe spirituality does not apply to atheists or agnostics

Strongly disagree   *Disagree*   *Uncertain*   *Agree*   *Strongly agree*
        *   *   *   *   *

q) I believe spirituality includes people's morals

Strongly disagree   *Disagree*   *Uncertain*   *Agree*   *Strongly agree*
        *   *   *   *   *

REFERENCES

Carson V B 1989 Spiritual dimensions of nursing practice. W B Saunders, Philadelphia

Emblen J D, Halstead L 1993 Spiritual needs and interventions: comparing the views of patients, nurses and chaplains. Clinical Nurse Specialist 7 (4): 175–182

Frankl V E 1987 Man's search for meaning. An introduction to logotherapy. Hodder & Stoughton, London

Harrison J, Burnard P 1993 Spirituality and nursing practice. Avebury, Aldershot

McSherry W 1997, A descriptive survey of nurses' perceptions of spirituality and spiritual care. Unpublished MPhil thesis, University of Hull, Hull

Narayanasamy A 1991 Spiritual care: a resource guide. Quay Books, Lancaster

Oppenheim A N 1992 Questionnaire design, interviewing and attitude measurement, new edn. Printer Publishers, London

Shelly J A, Fish S 1988 Spiritual care: the nurse's role, 3rd edn. Inter Varsity Press, Illinois

Waugh L A 1992 Spiritual aspects of nursing: a descriptive study of nurses' perceptions. Unpublished PhD thesis, Queen Margaret College, Edinburgh

Index